C0-AVN-706

# Clinical Ballistocardiography

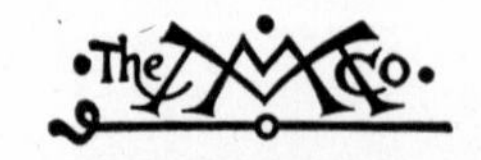

THE MACMILLAN COMPANY
NEW YORK • BOSTON • CHICAGO
DALLAS • ATLANTA • SAN FRANCISCO

MACMILLAN AND CO., LIMITED
LONDON • BOMBAY • CALCUTTA
MADRAS • MELBOURNE

THE MACMILLAN COMPANY
OF CANADA, LIMITED
TORONTO

# CLINICAL BALLISTOCARDIOGRAPHY

HERBERT R. BROWN, Jr., M.D.
VINCENT deLALLA, Jr., M.D.
MARVIN A. EPSTEIN, M.D.
MARVIN J. HOFFMAN, M.D.

*New York* *1952*
THE MACMILLAN COMPANY

First Printing, May, 1952.

*Printed in the United States of America*

*Dedicated to*

Ralph Hochstetter whose interest in the advances of medicine was both helpful and stimulating in this work

# FOREWORD

WIDESPREAD interest is being manifested in regard to new instrumentation in the study of the circulation of the blood. For a long time cardiologists were preoccupied with the study of electrical events occurring within the heart, and with the exploration of the diagnostic possibilities of the electrocardiogram, to such an extent that studies of the dynamics of the circulation as a whole languished. This preoccupation focused attention too exclusively upon the heart itself.

It is true that the heart is the prime mover of the circulation, initiating the pulse wave which progresses throughout the arterial tree expending much of its force against the peripheral resistance. How much of the blood expelled from the left ventricle in systole would find its way back to the right auricle if it were not for the assistance of the tonus of the muscles and the rhythmic movements of the respiratory apparatus which bring about reciprocal pressure changes between abdomen and thorax and which maintain the venous return to the right auricle?

The cardiac output and the force of the heart's systole are dependent upon the degree of diastolic filling with venous blood. A weak heartbeat does not necessarily imply a weak heart muscle; it may mean simply that there has been an inadequate supply of venous blood to distend it in diastole sufficiently to produce a strong systolic contraction, in accordance with Starling's law. Thus in the ballistocardiogram recoil movements of low amplitude may be formed when conditions in the peripheral circulation interfere with the venous return to a heart which may be fully capable of beating strongly. Hence we must be very careful not to think of this instrument in terms of the heart alone, but in terms of the circulation as a whole. It might have been better if it were simply called a ballistograph, omitting the "cardio" from the word.

Fortunately modern instrumentation makes possible the simultaneous recording of numerous events. The ballistic movements may be observed together with the electrocardiogram, ventilatory movements, and simultaneous pressure changes in pulmonic and systemic arteries under a wide variety of physiological conditions, so as to yield knowledge which would not be revealed by any single method of observation taken alone. In the period 1946–1952 during which the authors were working in the University of Rochester, the development of instrumentation in this field has been quite remarkable, particularly in regard to multichannel recorders. These have now attained a widespread commercial availability which makes possible the general use of the ballistocardiograph as a clinical tool. It is to be hoped that the premature introduction of highly simplified devices for recording body movements will not lead to misinterpretations which will bring discredit of the use of this potentially valuable tool as an instrument of considerable precision. In view of this possibility the reader is invited to give careful attention to the analysis of the physical characteristics of a good ballistocardiograph, which is ably presented herein.

It is characteristic of the new phase of development which medicine is entering that we are attempting to assess the adaptive responses of the organism as a whole to the stresses of the environment, and that we are beginning to take account of the pyschological milieu in which our patients live, as well as the milieu interne of their cells. Thus the ballistocardiograph may play its part in recording some of the circulatory events occurring during psychiatric interviews as aggressions are released, or when anxiety is aroused and hyperventilation occurs.

It would not be appropriate at this point to attempt a list of all the many uses for which this instrument may be employed. It is certain that its usefulness will be greatest if we do not regard it too narrowly as a diagnostic tool for the detection of organic heart lesions.

WILLIAM S. MCCANN, M.D.

## ACKNOWLEDGMENTS

THE aim of this book is to present essentially all of the pertinent data in the field of ballistocardiography as known today. It has been our purpose to gather the references and present them along with our findings, in a manner to which we have become accustomed to think. The entire field is young and concepts will change, but this does represent a starting point which we hope will facilitate the work of others interested in this type of cardiovascular study.

The authors wish to thank Dr. William S. McCann for his continuing advice, interest, and helpful suggestions from the very start of this work. We are also indebted to Dr. Harry A. Blair and Dr. Wallace O. Fenn for many helpful suggestions and criticisms as well as the actual construction of the table, which in this study was permanently borrowed from them. Credit is due to Dr. Raymond Pearson who contributed many suggestions which were helpful when this work first started. We appreciate the valuable help that Mr. Nat C. Jacobs rendered in the medical artistry preparation and mounting of figures. We wish also to thank Miss E. Elaine MacDowell who served as technician, subject, operator in the course of all of the experiments. Many thanks are given to Mrs. Cecilia A. Leib for her careful and repeated stenographic preparation of the manuscript. The abdominal supports used in the study of angina pectoris and sympathectomized patients were supplied by the Spencer Corset Company.

The entire work was greatly facilitated and the volume of study enhanced because of the support for a period of three years by the

Office of Naval Research, a research and development section of the United States Navy. This group provided the initial support and even when the work varied from the field of "Environmental Medicine" for which the original grant was made, this aid was still continued with almost all the emphasis being placed upon the ballistocardiograph in its experimental and clinical applications. The American Heart Association contributed aid in 1950 which was used to study the physical aspects of the ballistocardiograph apparatus itself. A continuing grant by the United States Public Health Service is now in effect allowing for further experimental work to continue, using the ballistocardiograph as an experimental instrument useful in the study of cardiovascular problems.

The authors are especially appreciative of the invaluable assistance of Mr. W. Holt Seale, editor-in-chief, and to Miss Barbara Russell, of the Medical Department of The Macmillan Company in the assemblage and preparation of the monograph itself.

HERBERT RUTHERFORD BROWN, JR.
VINCENT DELALLA, JR.
MARVIN ALLEN EPSTEIN
MARVIN JEROME HOFFMAN

Department of Medicine
University of Rochester
School of Medicine and Dentistry

January, 1952

# CONTENTS

## PART ONE

# NORMAL SECTION

PREFACE

# What Is the Ballistocardiogram and What Is Its Value?

THE term "ballistocardiogram" was originated by Starr in 1939 (*1*).* It is derived from the Greek: *ballein*—to throw; *kardia*—heart; *gramma*—a drawing. Literally, then, it means a drawing of the heart's throwing, or better, a record of the body movements produced by the heartbeat. Anyone can demonstrate this movement for himself by standing very still on a bathroom scale and observing the slight deflection of the pointer that takes place with each pulse. This movement, when magnified several thousand times and recorded, is a ballistocardiogram.

These movements have been known for almost 75 years and have been studied extensively for about 15 years. The earlier approach to the use of the waves was a quantitative one; i.e., the records were used almost exclusively for the calculation of cardiac output.

In the past 5 years the emphasis has included the qualitative aspects of the ballistocardiogram, with empirical analysis of patterns being carried on in several laboratories. As a result of these investigations ballistocardiography has demonstrated a real clinical usefulness. More and more workers have become interested in the field, and this monograph is designed as an aid to them and to those who have yet to

* Italic numbers in parentheses refer to the numbered list of published material appearing at the close of the chapter.

become engaged in this line of study. Routine clinical installations will be a reality in many places soon, and office installations are relatively inexpensive and practical for anyone with a direct-writing electrocardiograph.

This monograph will present a survey of the field from the theoretical and practical points of view, including the summarized findings of records made in our laboratory. This includes about 1,200 different subjects of whom 135 were considered normal clinically. As many as 40 tracings have been made serially in some patients, and the library consists of a total of nearly 3,000 records.

The basis for the clinical application of the ballistocardiogram is the well-documented fact that, in normal people, a repeatable pattern of waves occurs with every heartbeat. This is independent of the recording instrument but will vary with the mechanical device to which the body's motion is imparted. Starr used a wooden bed mounted on four strips of spring steel on a rugged wooden frame. These were arranged so that the bed could be displaced only in a headward and footward direction. The pickup translates the movement of the bed from mechanical displacement to an electrical signal. This in turn is fed into the recording instrument. Most of the information we have collected is based on this type of record.

Just what new information does the ballistocardiogram give us? The electrocardiogram records show the electrical potential changes occurring during the cardiac cycle, but the ballistocardiogram represents mechanical events and is more nearly related to the efficiency of heart action as a pump. The information is of value as a diagnostic tool and as a prognostic aid. It will be shown that the ballistocardiogram helps in the diagnosis of coronary disease, in the differentiation of uncomplicated hypertension from hypertensive heart disease, in the diagnosis of congestive heart failure, in the diagnosis of coarctation of the aorta, and in the determination of amount of recovery after myocardial infarction. Also, the ballistocardiogram has applications in public health and industrial medicine. Studies are not completed, but it is likely that long-term, large-scale investigations of employees will allow for the early diagnosis of subclinical heart or pulmonary disease, and the work evaluation of a partially disabled employee.

*Limitations*

The ballistocardiographic records are of little value in the following conditions:

1. When the heart rate is excessively rapid (140 or more).
2. When gross tremors or muscular tic are present.
3. When the individual (such as a semiconscious subject, or a very young child) is unco-operative and continually moves while on the table.
4. When there is great tachypnea.

Fortunately, these conditions are not frequently encountered.

## REFERENCE

### THE BALLISTOCARDIOGRAM AND ITS VALUE

1. Starr, I., Rawson, A. J., Schroeder, H. A., and Joseph, N. R.: "Studies on the Estimation of Cardiac Output in Man and of Abnormalities in Cardiac Function, from the Heart's Recoil and the Blood's Impact; the Ballistocardiogram," *Am. J. Physiol.*, **127**:1, 1939.

CHAPTER ONE

# The History of the Ballistocardiograph

---

THE modern ballistocardiograph is an adaptation of an old idea. J. W. Gordon (*1*) in 1877 first demonstrated that motion of the body occurs with each heartbeat. Gordon's observation that such motion exists is common to many people, and it is stated in his introductory remarks: "A person standing erect in a perfectly easy posture on the bed of an ordinary spring weighing machine, and maintaining, as far as possible, perfect stillness, will be found, if the instrument is delicately adjusted, to impart a rhythmic movement to the index, synchronous with the pulse . . . . It does not appear that this phenomenon has heretofore been anticipated by any process of theorizing, or turned to any useful account."

The first of two methods used by Gordon to derive a record from this motion was to allow the pointer of the weighing machine to trace out a figure. He later substituted a better device in the form of a light frame table suspended from a trestle by four ropes. The tracings obtained using these methods are reproduced in Figure 1. In theorizing as to the cause of these movements, Gordon felt that the vigorous downward movement of the mass of blood in the aorta and its accompanying recoil were responsible for the pulse waves which he noted to be synchronous with systole. A few years later (1880) Landois (*2*) described a simple and apparently effective vertical ballistocardiograph using Gordon's technique.

Further practical application has been made of the fact that certain types of scales show rhythmic deflections corresponding to the pulse

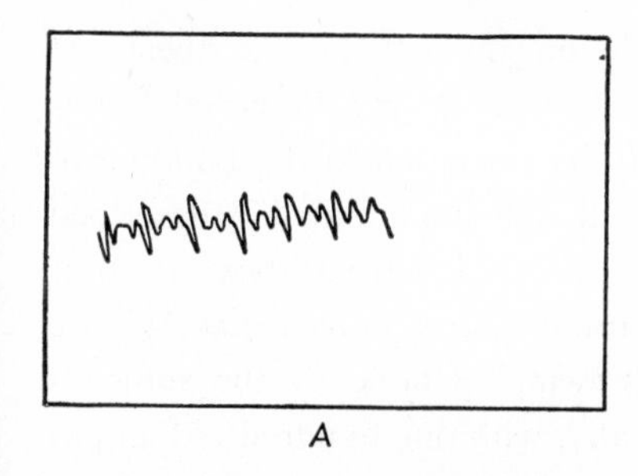


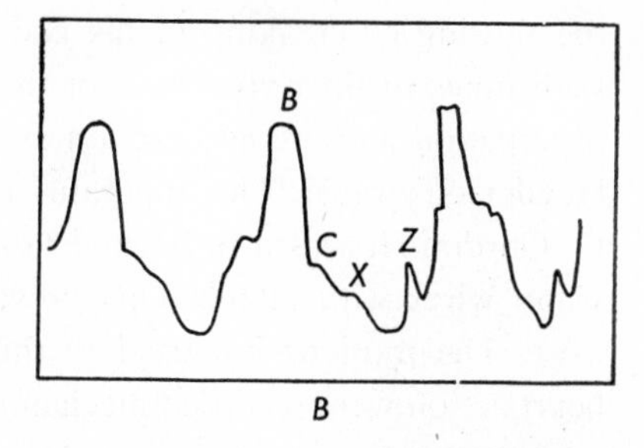


FIGURE 1. Pictures of Gordon's traces are shown. *A* was obtained from his weighing machine and *B* from a table suspended by ropes. In *A* the downstroke which is immediately succeeded by a long upstroke is synchronous with the systole; the next downstroke is the second deflection referred to by Gordon. The upstrokes are to be regarded merely as indicating the instrumental tendency to restore equilibrium. In *B* the letters bear the same significance as in Dr. Galabin's figures. *Vide infra.* (Gordon, J. W.: "On Certain Molar Movements of the Human Body Produced by the Circulation of the Blood," *J. Anat. & Physiol.,* **11**:533, 1877.)

of the subject being weighed. Seventy years later, Krahl, seeking a simple and inexpensive method for recording cardiac ballistics, made use of this observation in constructing a simple ballistocardiograph to be used as a teaching aid in the physiology laboratory (see Chapter 2).

Henderson (*3*) was next to experiment in this field. The aim of his investigation was to record the volume of the systolic discharge. In dogs the volume curve was obtained by enclosing the heart in a plethysmograph. Such a curve records the volume of each systolic discharge as well as the details of filling and emptying of the heart's chambers. The problem was to obtain similar information on human subjects under normal and pathological conditions. Cardiopneumograms, estimation of heart size from roentgenograms, and pulse pressure determinations from the newly developed sphygmomanometer were given consideration but discarded because of their limitations or impracticality. In 1905, a brief preliminary report was published by Henderson describing what he considered to be a new method for estimating the volume of blood moved by each heartbeat. He remarked that "on occasion most everyone has been kept awake by the rattling or creaking of his bed in unison with his heartbeat. At such times distinct vibrations of the entire body can be noted." This observation and a consideration as to its cause led to the building of Henderson's table. The apparatus used was similar to that described by Gordon. It was a horizontal table suspended from above by four piano wires with attachments preventing lateral movements (Figure 2A). The motions imparted to this swinging table by the subject's heart action were recorded mechanically, with one hundredfold ampli-

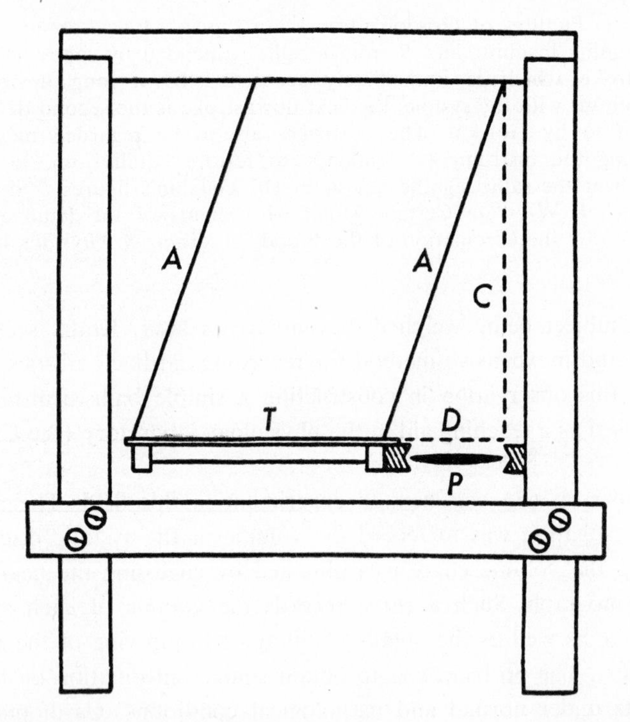


FIGURE 2A. Diagram of Henderson's table. A frame of heavy timbers was constructed somewhat like an old-fashioned four-poster bed. It is 2.0 meters long, 1.8 meters high, and 0.8 meter wide. One end is shown in the drawing. In this frame the swinging table *T* is suspended by four piano wires (*A, A*) fastened as shown, so that the motion is perpendicular to the plane of the drawing. The table itself is a thin plank 50 cm wide and 1.2 cm thick, supported and stiffened by stringers under each side connected by four cross pieces at equal intervals. It weighs 9 kg. At each

fication. Figure 2B is a reproduction of traces from Henderson's paper. Simultaneous carotid artery pulse records were made to indicate the relation to the cardiac cycle of the various features of the "Recoil Curve of the Circulation as a Whole," the name Henderson gave to the recorded pattern. He associated this "recoil curve" with the heart's action and the movement of blood in the great vessels. Newton's third law of motion (to every action there is an equal and opposite reaction) was thought to be applicable, hence the title "recoil curve." Henderson considered this "recoil curve" to be a quantitative expression of the algebraic sum of all the mass movements of the circulation.

In 1911, the Anglo-American Pikes Peak Expedition, reported by Douglas, Haldane, Henderson, and Schneider (*4*), made use of this

---

end of the table is a sharp-pointed steel pin *P*, 10 cm long and 2 mm thick. One end of each pin rests in a case-hardened steel cup sunk in the side of the table; the other end in a similar cup in the post of the frame. The latter pair of cups are adjustable in position both longitudinally and laterally. The use of these pins serves a double purpose. It limits the swinging table to longitudinal movements, the precise path of every point in the table being an arc of a circle whose radius is equal to the length of the pins. The second and more important object of the arrangement of the pins is to allow an adjustment of the table to a very slow pendulum swing. Thus, if the dotted line *C* represents a plumb line dropped from the origin of the wire *A*, and *D* the horizontal distance from the insertion of *A* to *C*, it is evident that only when *D* is shorter than (or at most just equal to) the length of the pin will the table rest in the position shown. As the steel cups in the frame are moved away from the table, its pendulum time is shortened; as they are moved out toward the table, the pendulum period is lengthened. Since the pins turn on their sharpened points with a minimum of friction, while the pendulum point can thus be lengthened almost to the vanishing point, the table not only moves under the influence of the slightest force (such as the flexing of a finger by the person lying upon it), but also remains stationary in the position at which it is brought to rest.

At each end of the table a stop is attached which by striking against the frame limits the total swing to 8 mm. Fastened to the frame at one end is a clutch by which the table is held motionless while the person to be examined is lying down or rising and until the respiratory movements have ceased.

(Henderson, Y.: "The Mass-Movements of the Circulation as Shown by a Recoil Curve," *Am. J. Physiol.,* **14**:287, 1905.)

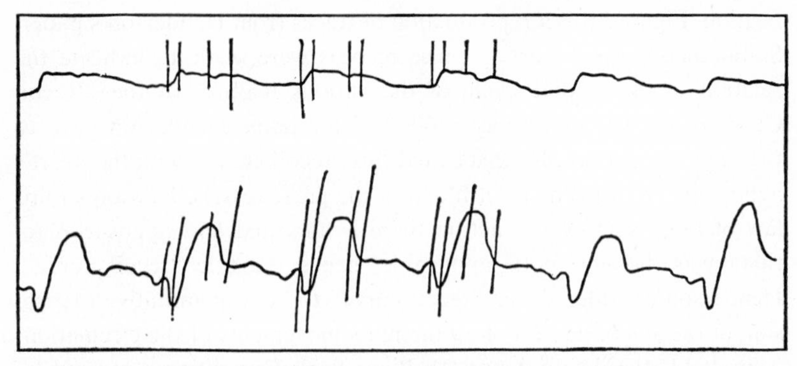

FIGURE 2B. Reproduction of the traces obtained from Henderson's table (lower traces in each group), correlated with the carotid pulsations (upper traces). (Henderson, Y.: "The Mass-Movements of the Circulation as Shown by a Recoil Curve," *Am. J. Physiol.,* **14**:287, 1905.)

recoil table in studying the effect of altitude on cardiac output. The apparatus used was a plank supported on rubber stoppers. It was found that the amplitude of the recorded pattern was practically the same on the peak as under ordinary barometric pressure, supporting a view that low barometric pressure per se does not alter the volume of systolic discharge. This is believed to be the first application of the ballistocardiograph in an acute experiment.

The next attempt to record body movements associated with mechanical systole did not take place until 1922. Heald and Tucker (*5*), having previously perfected the hot-wire microphone for military use, used it to record body motion as a means of measuring the efficiency of the heart. Their apparatus is pictured in Figure 3. It consists of two iron drums connected by a short piece of rubber tubing. The platform for the patient is suspended from a metal diaphragm which also is the base of the first drum. Movements of this base will send bursts of air through the tube to the second drum. The hot-wire microphone is placed between the tubing and the second drum; it is cooled by the bursts of air, thereby diminishing its electrical resistance. These changes in resistance unbalance a Wheatstone bridge, causing deflection of a string galvanometer. The ohmmeter allows for standardization of sensitivity and also for quantitative comparison of records.

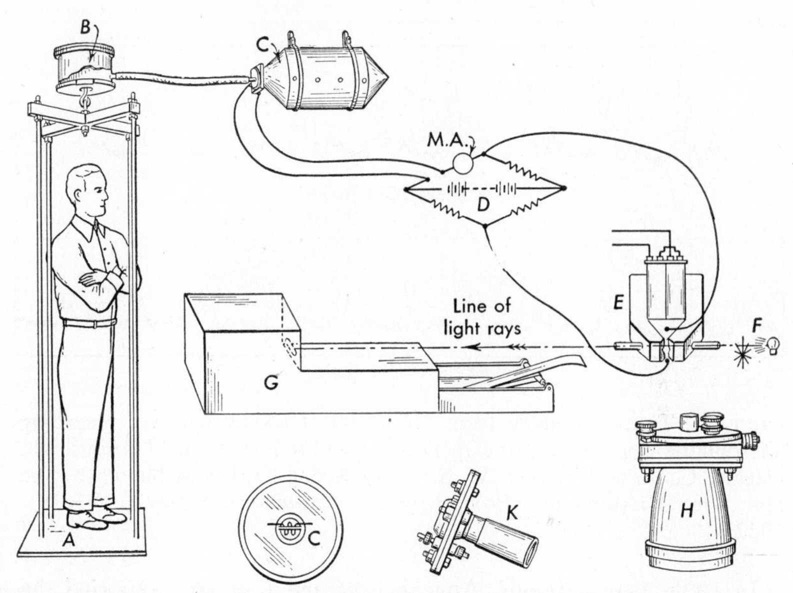


FIGURE 3. Heald and Tucker's hot-wire recording apparatus. (*A*) Platform, (*B*) drum and diaphragm, (*C*) microphone and accessory cylinder, ($C^1$) microphone grid, (*D*) Wheatstone bridge circuit, (*E*) Einthoven galvanometer, (*F*) source of light and time wheel, (*G*) camera and automatic developer, (*H*) pulse microphone, (*K*) breathing microphone. (Heald, C. B., and Tucker, W. S.: "The Recoil Curves as Shown by the Hot Wire Microphone," *Proc. Roy. Soc. (London),* Series B, **93**:281, 1922.)

The tracings obtained by this method were excellent (Figure 4), although only positive deflections were recorded since all movements of air, whether in or out, cooled the grid of the microphone. It was shown that correcting for these negative deflections by reversing alternating peaks produced tracings very similar to those of Henderson. After mathematical analysis the records were considered to measure quantities related to the kinetic energy imparted to the body by motion of the blood. Besides showing this method to be effective for assaying cardiac function, Heald and Tucker demonstrated greater amplitude of the complexes during inspiration, attributing this change to normal physiological variations in cardiac output during respiration. This respiratory variation has assumed considerable importance in recent ballistocardiography.

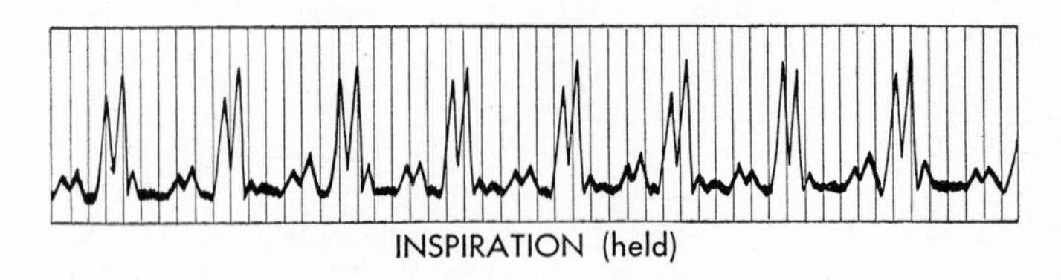


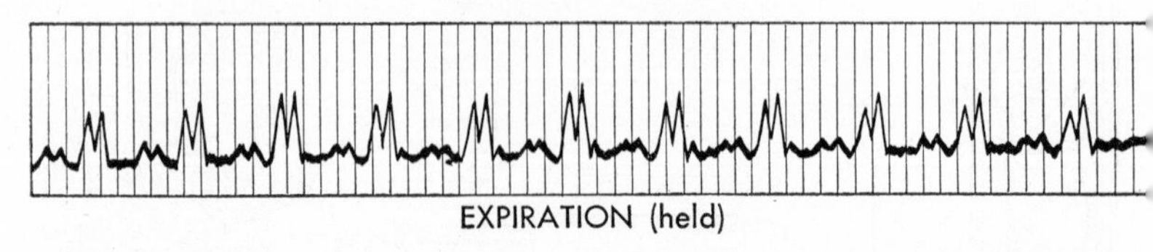


FIGURE 4. Traces obtained from Heald and Tucker's hot-wire recording microphone apparatus. Note increased amplitude with held inspiration. (Heald, C. B., and Tucker, W. S.: "The Recoil Curves as Shown by the Hot Wire Microphone," *Proc. Roy. Soc. (London),* Series B, **93**:281, 1922.)

In 1928, two Germans, Angenheister and Lau (*6*), reported the use of a seismograph in recording the movements caused by heart action. The subject lies on a firm, short-legged table as shown in Figure 5. The seismograph is placed on this table, while the recording

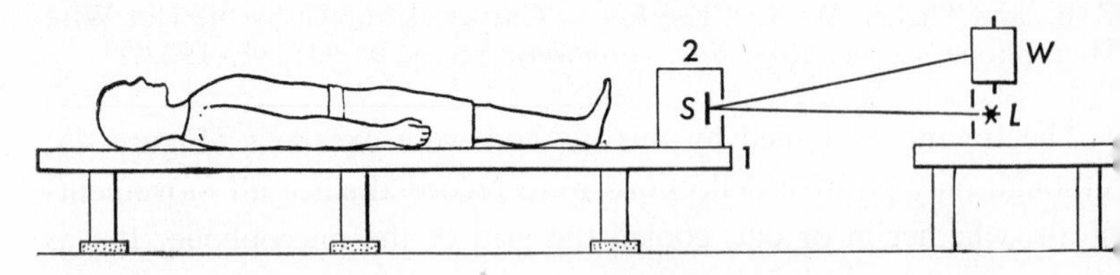


FIGURE 5. A drawing of the apparatus of Angenheister and Lau. The subject and seismograph (*S*) are placed on a firm table with short legs; the recording apparatus is on another table 1 meter away. The impulse created by the heart action is transferred to the table and seismograph and then recorded by optical means. (Angenheister, G., and Lau, E.: "Seismographische Aufnahmen der Hertztatigkeit," *Naturwissenschaften,* **16**:513, 1928.)

apparatus rests on a table 1 meter away. The impulse created by the heart action is transferred to the table and seismograph and optically registered. Figure 6 shows tracings obtained by this method.

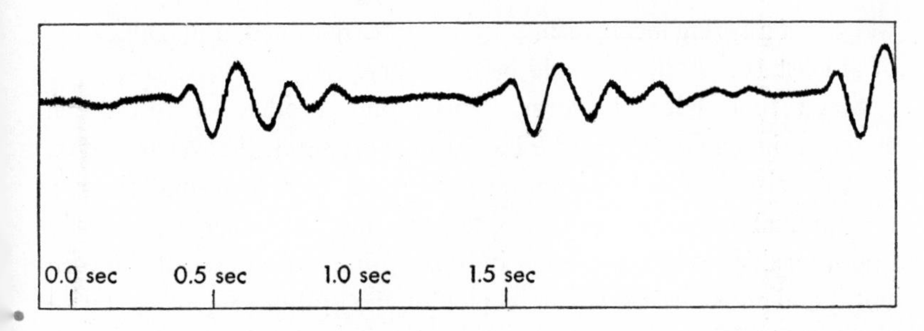


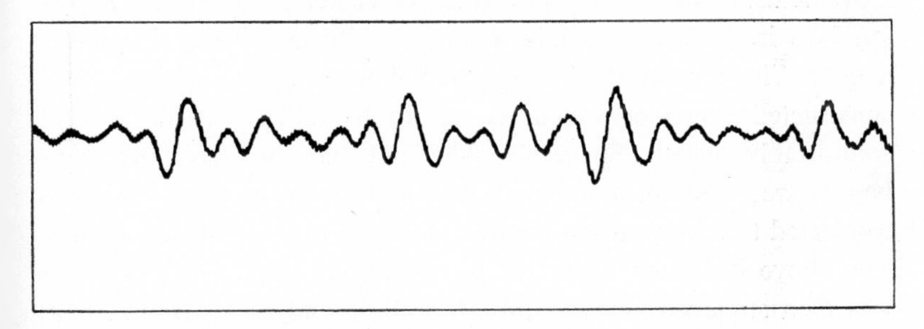

FIGURE 6. Traces obtained from the apparatus of Angenheister and Lau. Note the presence of after waves. (Angenheister, G., and Lau, E.: "Seismographische Aufnahmen der Herztatigkeit," *Naturwissenschaften,* **16**:513, 1928.)

A Swedish physiologist, Abramson (7), was aware of this work and was very much interested in it. He too desired to record the movements of the body associated with each heartbeat. Abramson, however, was the first to apply physical principles in considering this problem. As a result of his calculations he at first thought the machine that would give him the exactness he sought could not be made, since it would require too much magnification. He desired the frequency response of the apparatus to be at least 50 vibrations per second. Presumably, this minimum requirement was based on Otto Frank's principle that the vibrating frequency of the recording apparatus must be kept far away from the frequency to be recorded if a true response is to be obtained. Ordinarily, this can be accomplished by reducing to a minimum the mass of the system to be measured, but in this instance the lower margin of the mass is determined by the body weight. If a spring mechanism were used, he reasoned, a magnification of at least 10,000 times would be necessary.

Some time later, however, Abramson's brother, a Stockholm engineer, invented a device for measuring very small changes in length. This consisted of a blade spring which was turned around its own longitudinal axis, one half to one side and the other half to the opposite side. When the ends of this spring are stretched between static and movable parts, the center of the spring executes rotating movements. With a mirror placed in the center of the spring, a very sensitive instrument is obtained for optically measuring changes in length. With the problem of magnification solved, a scale was then constructed which permitted records to be taken with the patient comfortably seated (Figure 7). The movable part (seat and foot-board) was made of aluminum alloy to decrease its mass. This was connected to a very strong pig-iron stand by two hard blade springs. The above described apparatus for measuring small length changes was then stretched between this static base and the movable chair, with a screw adjustment permitting changes in tension and in the position of the mirror. This excellently constructed instrument had a natural frequency of 148 cycles per second when empty and a frequency response of 75 cycles per second with a 70-kg load. With the camera 1 meter away, the magnification was approximately 130,000:1.

The records obtained with this well-designed apparatus were called "kardiodynamograms" (Figure 8). These were considered impulse force diagrams related to the acceleration the heart action gives to part of the blood volume as well as to its own mass; i.e., they are an expression of motion change.

A great deal of credit is due Abramson for his work. He not only demonstrated the usefulness of a spring mechanism in constructing a suitable apparatus, but he was the first to give theoretical as well as empirical consideration to the kardiodynamogram. He developed a formula with which he hoped to calculate minute volume and planned to make a comparison with the Grollman acetylene method and possibly obtain a correlation constant for the formula. Starr (*8*) found this formula for cardiac output to be erroneous, but he expressed regret that Abramson did not continue with his proposed experiments.

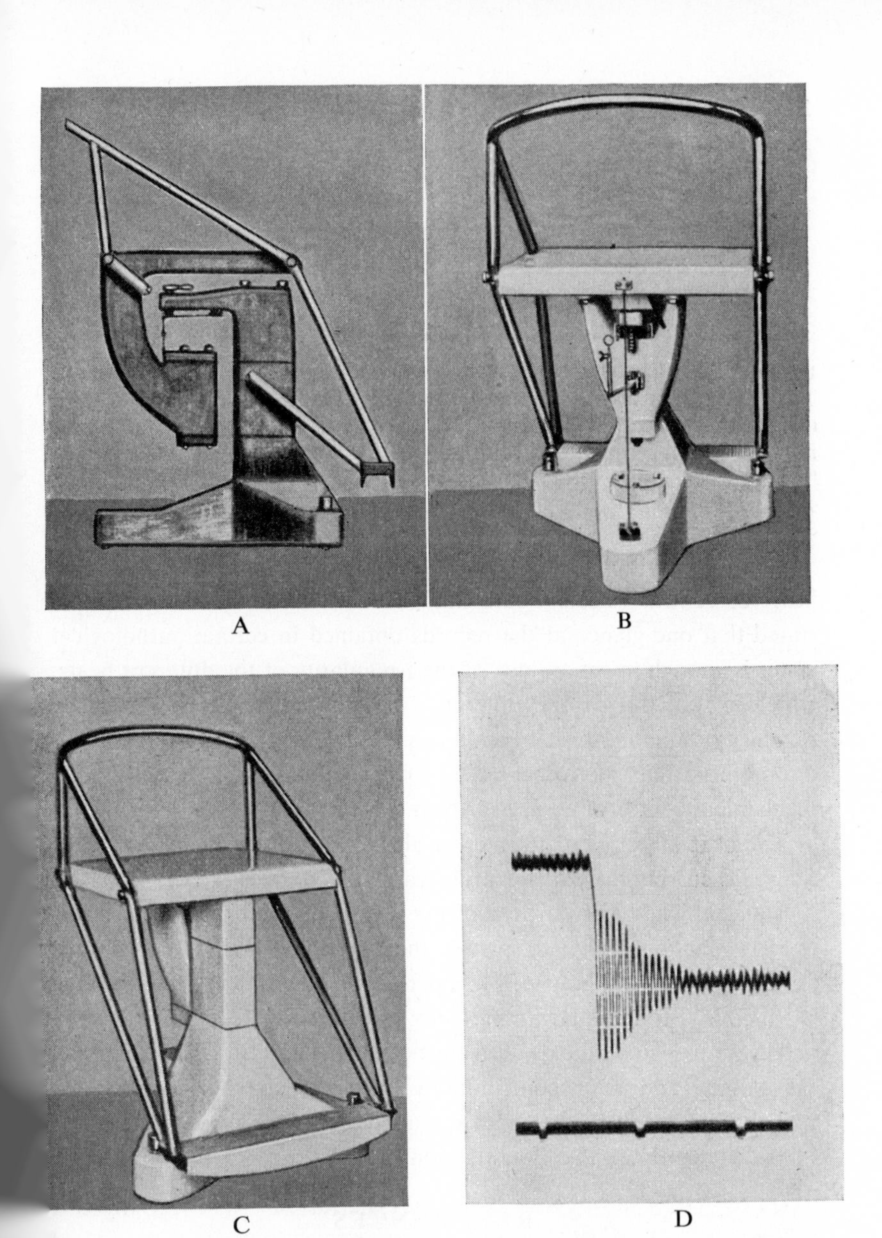


FIGURE 7. *A, B,* and *C* are pictures of Abramson's apparatus which is in the form of a chair and allows the subject to be comfortably seated while the trace is obtained. *D* is a trace of the natural frequency obtained with this apparatus, when loaded with 70 kg of dead weight. (Abramson, E.: "Die Rückstosskurve des Herzens (Kardiodynamogramm)," *Skandinav. Arch. f. Physiol.,* **66**:191, 1933.)

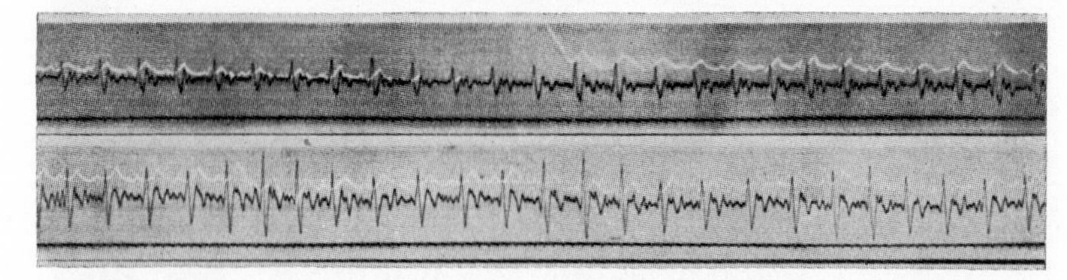

FIGURE 8. The traces pictured are those obtained by Abramson's apparatus. The top trace is a control; the bottom trace was taken 30 minutes after the administration of Adrenalin (0.7 mg). Note that the after waves are not simple oscillations returning to the base line. (Abramson, E.: "Die Rückstosskurve des Herzens (Kardiodynamogramm)," *Skandinav. Arch. f. Physiol.*, **66**:191, 1933.)

Abramson anticipated that certain pathological conditions of the heart or central vessels would influence the kardiodynamogram. He stated that one glance at the records obtained in certain pathological states is enough to get an idea of the irregularity of the different beats, which is something quite different from the constant, characteristic regularity found in normal conditions. He felt that the kardiodynamogram (more than any other method) makes it possible to follow the mechanical course of each heartbeat.

The next investigator to interest himself in this problem was Isaac Starr. Discussing the ballistocardiograph in *The Harvey Lectures* (9), he stated: "The chief purpose of my investigations has been a simple one. I want to be able to answer the question whether the heart is strong or weak, and how well it is performing the function of pumping the blood." From the beginning Starr and his co-workers have investigated the ballistocardiograph from both the theoretical and empirical viewpoints, and their contributions have been numerous and significant—so much so that with the advent of Starr's work a new era of ballistocardiographic investigation began.

## REFERENCES

### HISTORY

1. GORDON, J. W.: "On Certain Molar Movements of the Human Body Produced by the Circulation of the Blood," *J. Anat. & Physiol.*, **11**:533, 1877.

2. LANDOIS, L.: *Lehrbuch der Physiologie des Menschen,* Vienna, 1880. (Quoted by Lamport, H.: *Science,* **93**:305, 1941.)
3. HENDERSON, Y.: "The Mass-Movements of the Circulation as Shown by a Recoil Curve," *Am. J. Physiol.,* **14**:287, 1905.
4. DOUGLAS, C. G., HALDANE, J. S., HENDERSON, Y., and SCHNEIDER, E. C.: "VI. Physiological Observations Made on Pike's Peak, Colorado, with Special Reference to Adaptation to Low Barometric Pressures," *Trans. Roy. Soc. (London),* Series *B,* **203**:185, 1913.
5. HEALD, C. B., and TUCKER, W. S.: "The Recoil Curves as Shown by the Hot Wire Microphone," *Proc. Roy. Soc. (London),* Series *B,* **93**:281, 1922.
6. ANGENHEISTER, G., and LAU, E.: "Seismographische Aufnahmen der Herztatigkeit," *Naturwissenschaften,* **16**:513, 1928.
7. ABRAMSON, E.: "Die Rückstosskurve des Herzens (Kardiodynamogramm)," *Skandinav. Arch. f. Physiol.,* **66**:191, 1933.
8. STARR, I., RAWSON, A. J., SCHROEDER, H. A., and JOSEPH, N. R.: "Studies on the Estimation of Cardiac Output in Man, and of Abnormalities in Cardiac Function, from the Heart's Recoil and the Blood's Impacts; the Ballistocardiogram," *Am. J. Physiol.,* **127**:1, 1939.
9. STARR, I.: "The Ballistocardiograph—an Instrument for Clinical Research and for Routine Clinical Diagnosis," *Harvey Lect.,* 1946–1947, Series 42, The Science Press, Lancaster, Pa., p. 194.

## CHAPTER TWO

# Types of Apparatus Used in Recording the Ballistocardiogram

---

THE types of apparatus used in obtaining ballistocardiograms vary in their frequency response and structure. This chapter will present brief descriptions and discussions of the various kinds of modern instruments. With the growing interest in this field commercial production of several types of instruments began. The reasons for our selection of a high frequency type of table are given in Chapter 3, and the physicists who developed the commercial types of apparatus have felt similarly, as may be seen in the description of design and instrument construction. It has been convenient to compare the records obtained by us and reproduced in this monograph. It can be added that the records obtained by the instruments to be discussed, irrespective of their type, are reasonably comparable to those obtained by the Starr-type table.

### The Horizontal Undamped "High-frequency" Table

Isaac Starr, in 1939, first used the term "ballistocardiograph," and it was his stimulating work which has lent considerable impetus to investigators in this field (*1*). The table which Starr developed is pictured in Figure 9. It consists of a thin panel of plywood mounted on a spruce frame, suspended from the ceiling by four steel wires.

ateral motion of the table is prevented by two braces attached to the arby wall and thence to the table through a flexible joint so that no sistance is offered to longitudinal motion (Figure 9). An adjustable

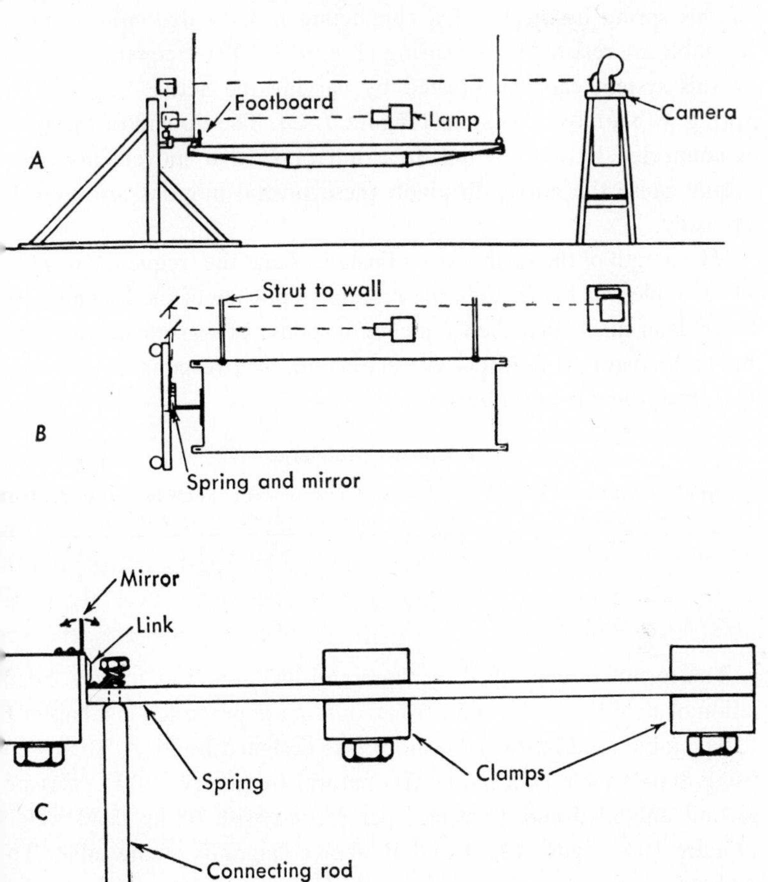


IGURE 9. Starr's original ballistocardiograph apparatus. From the side nd above. Details of spring and mirror; the left clamp may be moved long the spring to change its characteristics. Pushed about 3 in. from ts center of balance, the suspended table rests against the spring. (Starr, ., Rawson, A. J., Schroeder, H. A., and Joseph, N. R.: "Studies on the Estimation of Cardiac Output in Man, and of Abnormalities in Cardiac Function, from the Heart's Recoil and the Blood's Impact; the Ballisto-cardiogram," *Am. J. Physiol.,* **127**:1, 1939.)

spring of hardened tool steel ⅛ in. thick and ¾ in. wide is mounte on a rigid welded-steel structure made of pipe which is screwed to th floor and braced against the wall. The table is clamped to one en of this spring by means of a connecting rod, so that movements ( the table are resisted by the spring (Figure 9). The frequency respons of this system can be adjusted by varying the active length of th spring with a movable clamp (Figure 9, *C*). The tip end of the sprin is connected by a short link to a mirror so that movements of th spring cause the mirror to pivot; these pivotal motions are recorde optically.

The length of the spring was adjusted so that the frequency respons of the table was higher than the natural frequency of the human body Starr determined that the frequency response of warm cadavers upo his table averaged 5.76 cycles per second. The response of the tabl to a fixed force is as follows:

**Frequency Response**

| *Weight Added to Table, Pounds* | *Frequency Response, Cycles per Second, after Applying Stimulus to Table's End* |
|---|---|
| 50 | 15.5 |
| 100 | 12.5 |
| 150 | 10.5 |
| 200 | 9.5 |

The formulae developed by Starr and his associates for the calcu lation of stroke volumes and cardiac output are presented in Chapter 6

The table used in this laboratory was designed by H. A. Blair (*2*) using Starr's table as a model. Its natural frequency is 32 cycles pe second unloaded and 15 cycles per second with 68-kg dead weigh (Figure 10). Figure 11, *A* and *B*, shows diagrams of the table. Th table top is made of ⅞-in. plywood. This is mounted on four strip of stiff spring steel which are fixed to a heavy base made from 6-in by 6-in. fir timbers with crossbars for rigidity. The four springs ar placed equidistantly from the ends of the table top along both longi tudinal sides, so that only longitudinal motion is possible. These springs are made of high-carbon steel. Their dimensions and the de tails of their positioning can be found in Figure 12. The frequency o the table can be varied by changing the active length of the springs

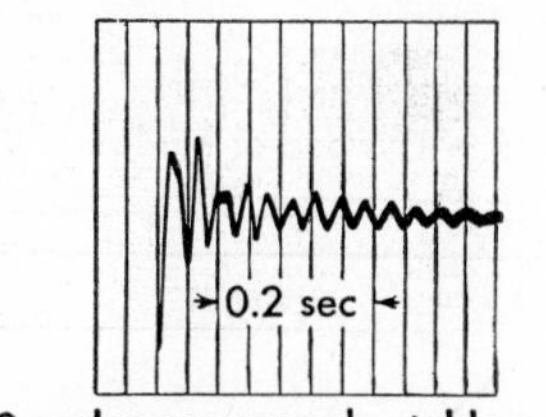


32 cycles per second – table empty

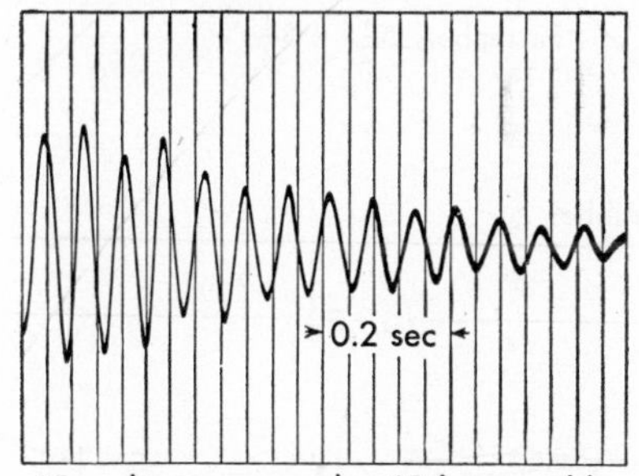


15 cycles per second – 68 kg on table

FIGURE 10. Frequency response of the Starr-type table used in our laboratory. The upper figure shows the response when the table is empty and the lower one with 68-kg dead weight on the table.

The records obtained from Starr's table and similar tables are force traces. It was decided to use Starr's table since the large library of Starr's records could thus be compared with those obtained by our apparatus, and since, in our present opinion, a high-frequency table is preferable to a low-frequency table (see below).

Dugald Brown (*3*) designed a portable horizontal table, using the same general principles as did Starr. Figure 13 shows a diagram of this table, taken from his article.

### *The Technitrol Horizontal Ballistocardiograph*

The Technitrol horizontal ballistocardiograph (Figure 14) is of the Starr type and consists of a vibrating bed of aluminum construction, weighing approximately 27 lb, freely suspended in a heavy steel-pipe frame weighing approximately 135 lb. (It is made by the Technitrol Engineering Company, Philadelphia, Pa.) The freedom

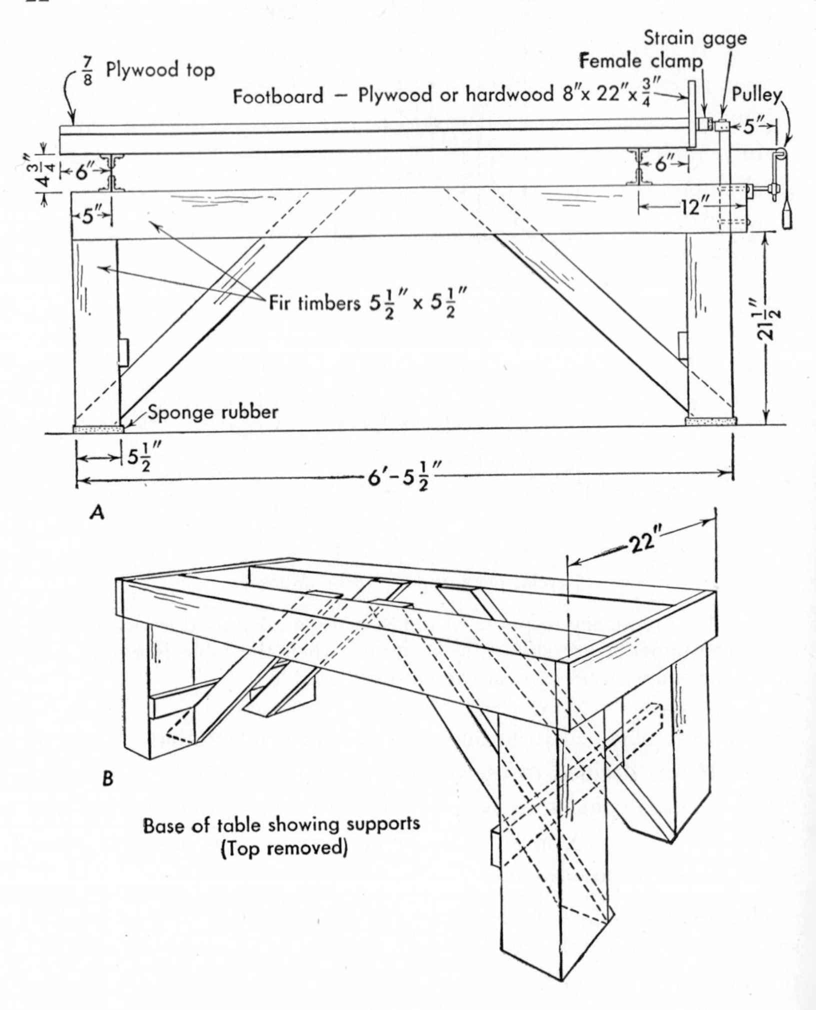


FIGURE 11. *A* and *B* are diagrams of the table in use in our laboratory.

of motion of the bed is restrained by a stiff leaf spring rigidly supported in the frame. This spring is stiff enough so that when the bed is loaded with 160-lb solid weight, the natural frequency is above 13 cycles per second. Under these conditions the amount of damping when unloaded or loaded with a rigid weight is quite small.

The bed-and-frame unit is 6 ft 8 in. long by 21 in. wide by 33 in high. It is equipped with large rubber casters for ease of moving. Four extension feet operated by knobs are provided to lift the unit from the casters and to level it. The vibration pickup and amplifier are mounted inside the frame under one end of the bed where the calibration weight and controls are located. The complete unit is finished in a hard, durable "Hammertone" finish which is impervious to most solvents and is easily kept clean.

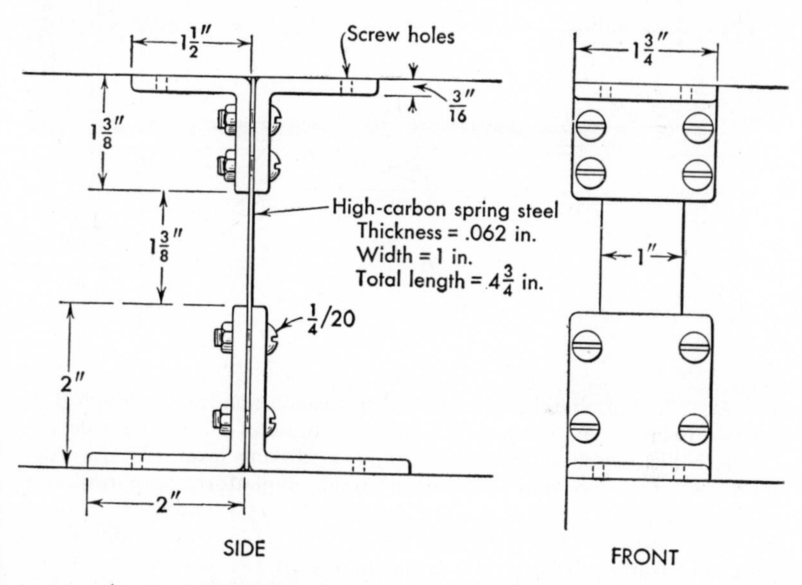


FIGURE 12. The dimensions and details of the spring mountings for the ballistocardiograph table used in this laboratory.

The vibration pickup unit is placed so as to pick up the relative motion between the bed and frame. The pickup is built up around the R.C.A. 5734 mechano-electro transducer tube which converts mechanical motion into an electrical signal. This signal is amplified to sufficient level to drive the recorder mechanism. The amplifier frequency response is flat from zero to several thousand cycles per second. The pickup-unit frequency response is flat to over 200 cycles per second. With direct-recording instruments frequency response is flat to 50 to 70 cycles per second. With string- and mirror-galva-

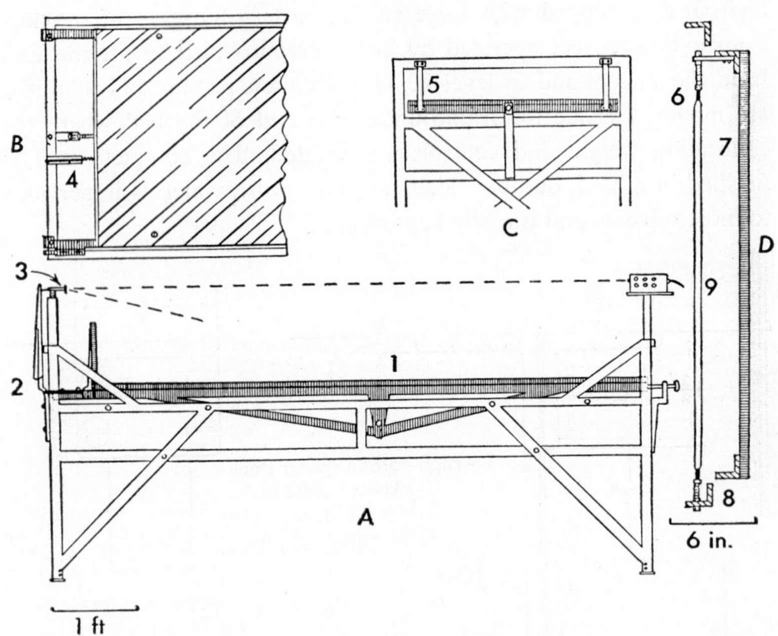


FIGURE 13. Portable horizontal ballistocardiograph table designed by Dugald Brown using the same principles as those of Starr. (*A*) Side view of the ballistograph showing platform (*1*), driving lever (*2*), recording lever (*3*); (*B*) top view, showing position of platform with respect to frame and position of calibrating spring (*4*); (*C*) end view, showing platform suspended by spring steel strips (*5*); (*D*) cross section of platform and frame, showing arrangement of strut (*9*) between frame (*8*) and platform (*7*), thereby preventing lateral movement. At either end, the ⅜-in. strut is connected to the platform and frame, respectively, by a strip of spring steel ½ in. by 1/32 in. (Brown, D. E.: "The Design of the Ballistocardiograph," *J. Clin. Investigation,* **21**:294, 1942.)

nometer-type recorders, much higher frequency responses are available.

The ballistocardiograph is designed for operation on 115 to 120 volts, 60 cycles per second, alternating current. The power cord is provided with a third wire for grounding purposes. In order to protect operators and subjects from the possibility of electrical shock, this third wire should be grounded to the building's electrical ground, i.e., a water pipe or the mounting screw in the wall plug.

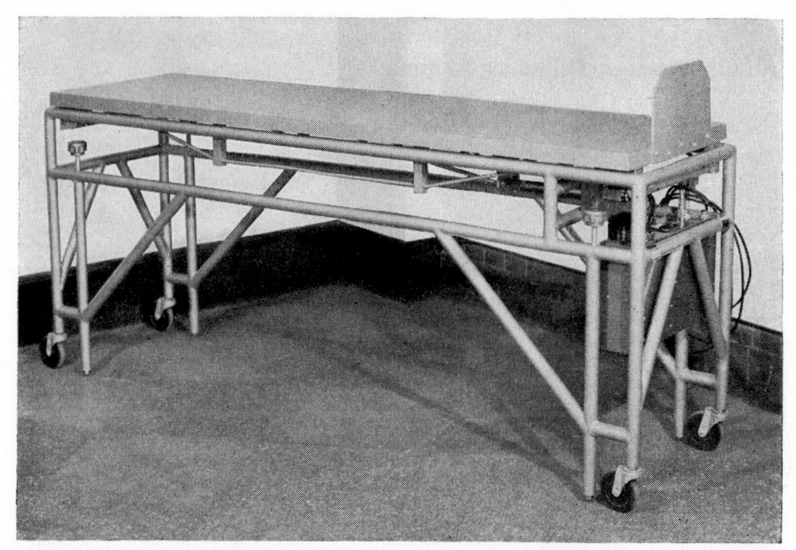

FIGURE 14. The Technitrol horizontal ballistocardiograph. This is an instrument made of steel. It is raised from casters and rests on four sturdy adjusted steel legs while the records are being taken. Any direct-writing electronic recording system of direct-coupled type may be used to direct the output signal from the "vibration pickup" which is a mechano-electro transducer tube converting mechanical motion into an electrical signal. (Courtesy of the Technitrol Engineering Company.)

Before using it, the instrument should be raised from the casters and leveled by means of the four leveling knobs on the frame. The ropes used for bracing the bed in shipment should be removed.

The ballistocardiograph is calibrated by applying a horizontal force to the bed and noting the deflection of the recorder. Standard practice has been to have 280 gm give 1-cm deflection. This will be approximately the case with the sensitivity control set at 0. To increase the sensitivity this control should be turned counterclockwise. It will be noted that the zero will shift as the sensitivity is increased or decreased. This shift should be corrected by adjustment of the vibration pickup knob. The calibrating unit will apply this force to the bed when the 8-oz weight is hung from the horizontal arm. When not in use, the calibrating weight can be removed and the lever flipped back to rest under the bed.

## Critically Damped Ballistocardiograph

Nickerson (*4*) and his co-workers developed a low-frequency critically damped ballistocardiograph, which is shown and described in Figure 15. This type of table employs weak springs and critical

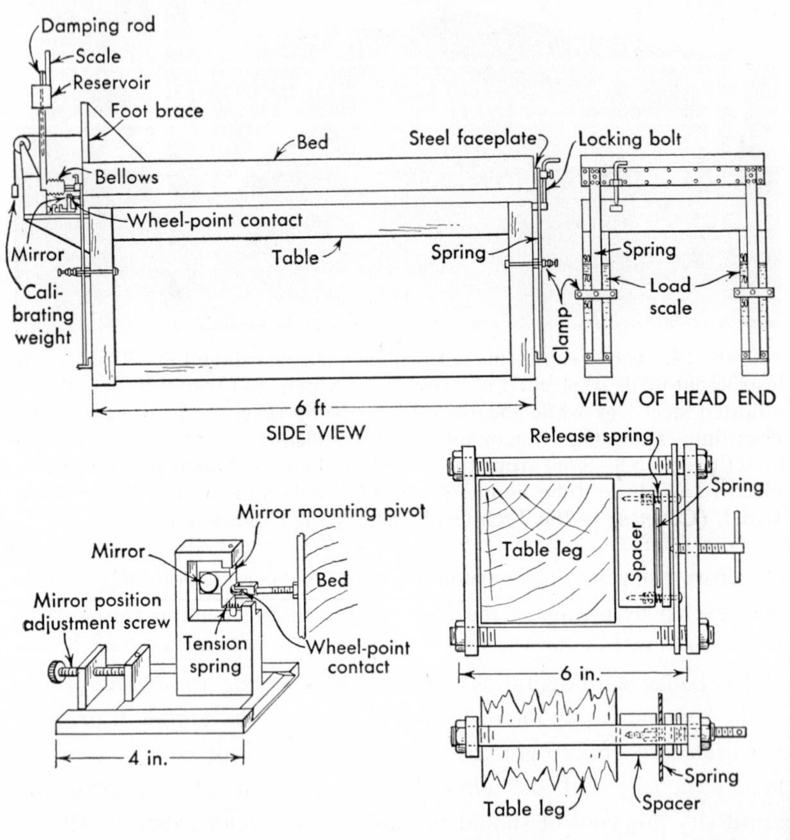


FIGURE 15. Nickerson's low-frequency critically damped table. Details of the construction of the ballistic bed as mounted on a table. The figure shows the flat springs on which the bed is supported, the spring clamps, the locking bolt, the damping system, the pickup mirror mounting, and wheel-point contact. The spring clamp and mirror system are shown in considerable detail. (Nickerson, J. L., Warren, J. W., and Brannon, E. S.: "The Cardiac Output in Man; Studies with the Low Frequency, Critically-damped Ballistocardiograph, and the Method of Right Atrial Catheterization," *J. Clin. Investigation,* **26**:1, 1947.)

damping so that the frequency response is held to approximately 1.5 cycles per second with the subject on the table. This is desired so that there will be no interference with the true amplitude of the IJ stroke by forces occurring at the onset of the cardiac cycle. The type of pattern obtained is shown in Figure 16. The theoretical disadvantages

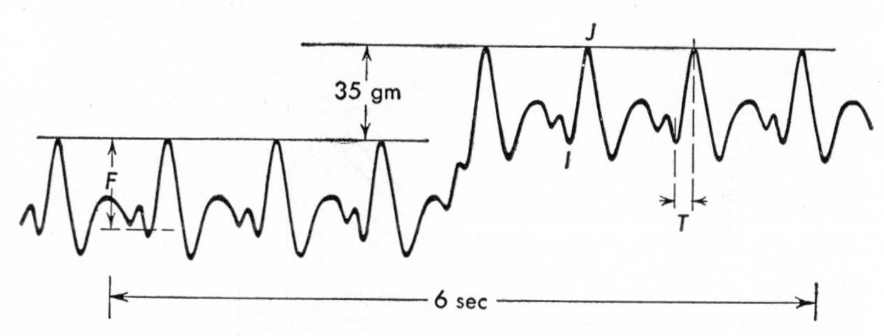


FIGURE 16. Ballistocardiogram taken with Nickerson's low-frequency damped table. The letters *F, I, J,* and *T* refer to the formula of Nickerson. A characteristic ballistocardiograph record, this demonstrates the method of calibration and indicates the measurements to be taken from the tracing. (Nickerson, J. L., Warren, J. W., and Brannon, E. S.: "The Cardiac Output in Man; Studies with the Low Frenquency, Critically-damped Ballistocardiograph, and the Method of Right Atrial Catheterization," *J. Clin. Investigation,* **26**:1, 1947.)

of the low-frequency critically damped ballistocardiograph are discussed below.

### The Vertical Ballistocardiograph

In 1941, Starr and Rawson (5) developed a vertical ballistocardiograph of light weight. A duraluminum platform was attached to a vertical steel frame which, in turn, was flexibly connected to a heavy steel-base frame, so that the platform could move only in a vertical direction. The vertical movement was resisted by two stiff, flat, steel springs, the tension of which could be adjusted by altering the active length (Figure 17). Relative movement between the platform and base drives a mirror mounted on a short lever, thus deflecting a light beam. This deflection was recorded on a standard photokymograph.

In order to obtain records free from vertical building vibrations it was necessary to weight the base with 500 lb of steel and to support

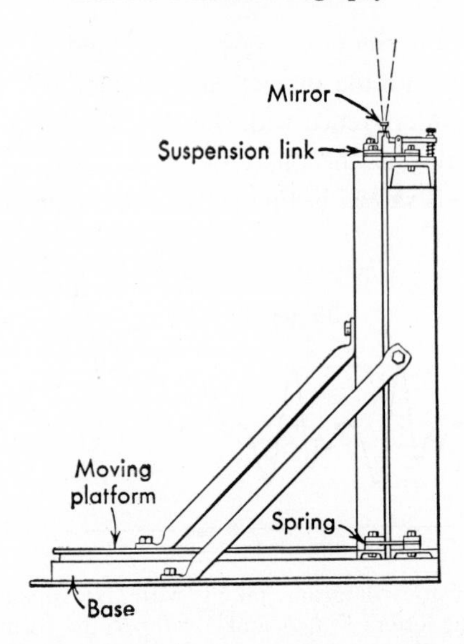


FIGURE 17. Illustrations of the vertical ballistocardiograph table of Starr and Rawson. (Starr, I., and Rawson, A. J.: "The Vertical Ballistocardiograph: Experiments on the Changes in the Circulation on Arising: with a Further Study of Ballistic Theory," *Am. J. Physiol.,* **134**:403, 1941.)

the entire mechanism on elastic material of diverse properties. The springs of the instrument were adjusted so that 280 gm placed on the platform caused a l-cm displacement on the record.

When weighted with varying weights and struck a single blow, the frequency was as follows:

| *Weight Added, Pounds* | *Frequency Response, Vibrations per Second* |
|---|---|
| 100 | 22 |
| 180 | 11.5 |
| 200 | 10.5 |

The frequency of this vertical instrument is almost 80 per cent greater than the horizontal at 100 lb, but only 10 per cent greater at 200 lb of added weight.

Perhaps the simplest vertical ballistocardiograph was described by Krahl (*6*). This consisted of an ordinary spring bathroom scale, a lever arrangement, and a kymograph drum (Figure 18). The deflec-

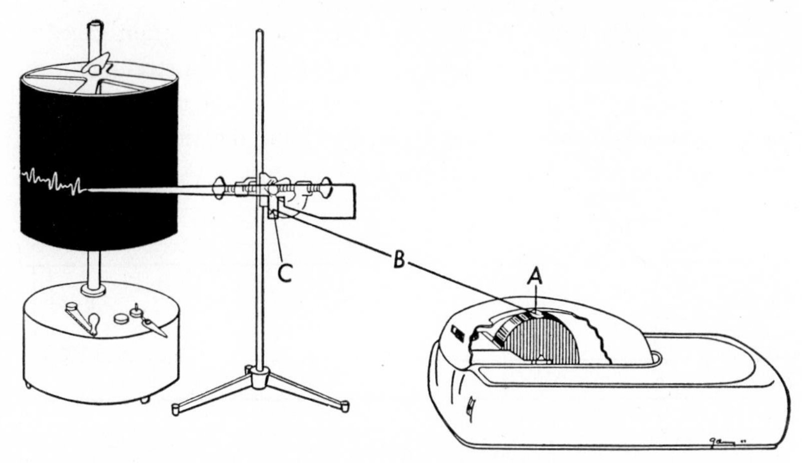


FIGURE 18. Krahl's simple vertical ballistocardiograph. (*A*) Detecto scale with a stiff wire (*B*) attached to the drum of the scale at *A*. The other end of the wire engages in a small hole in the writing lever at *C*. The lever is cut from a thin sheet of celluloid. A conventional type of kymograph is used for the recording apparatus. To obtain the record the subject stands upon the scale and when the scale mechanism has reached its equilibrium, the wire is attached to the drum at one end and to the lever at the other. (Krahl, V. E.: "A Simple Laboratory Apparatus for Demonstration of Cardiac Ballistics," *Science,* **105**:393, 1947.)

tions of the scale were transmitted by means of a rigid wire to the short end of a balanced lever. The long end of the lever wrote directly on a smoked kymograph drum. The sensitivity could be varied by adjusting the point of attachment of the rigid wire in relation to the fulcrum of the lever. The records obtained are satisfactory and useful for classroom demonstration (Figure 19).

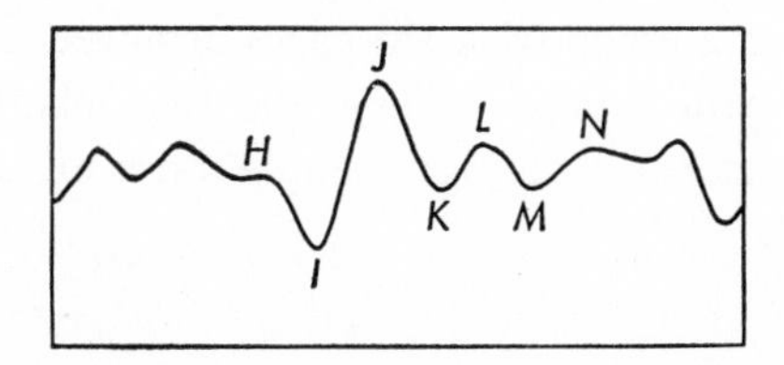


FIGURE 19. Trace obtained by the scale vertical ballistocardiograph pictured in Figure 18. Typical pattern with the waves indicated by the customary letters. (Krahl, V. E.: "A Simple Laboratory Apparatus for Demonstration of Cardiac Ballistics," *Science,* **105**:393, 1947.)

More recently Krahl (*7*) has described the use of strain gages to record the vertical impacts of subjects standing upon a steel platform. The dimensions of the strain-gage ballistocardiograph and its carrying case are approximately 3 in. by 16 in. by 18 in.; the apparatus weighs 30 lb including the 18-lb steel platform (Figure 20A). Figure 20B

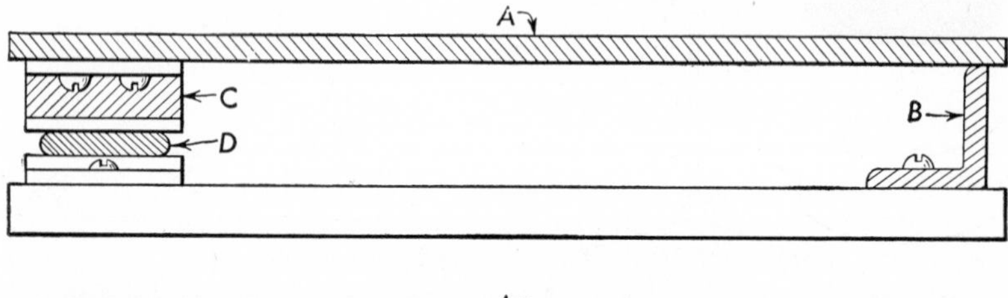


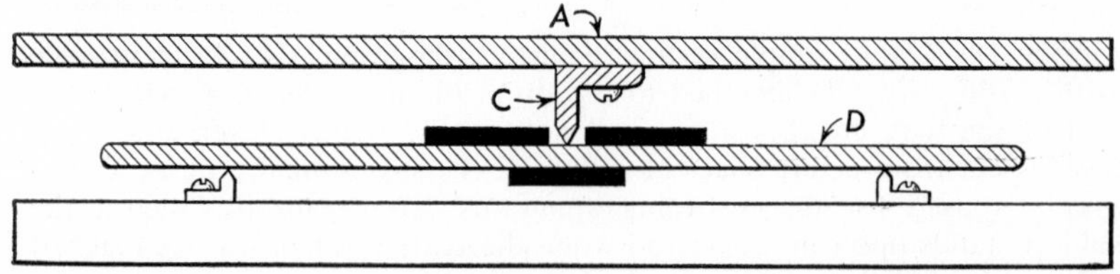


FIGURE 20A. Krahl's electric-strain-gage ballistocardiograph, side and front views. (*A*) Steel plate, ¼ in. by 14 in. by 14 in.; (*B*) 1-in. angle iron supporting one edge of the platform; (*C*) angle iron with sharpened edge, bolted to the center of the opposite edge; (*D*) steel recording bar, 3/16 in. by 1½ in. by 10 in., supported on the sharpened edges of two small angle irons and having a free length of 7½ in. Solid black strips on the recording bar indicate the position of the strain gages. (Krahl, V. E.: "The Electric Strain Gauge Ballistocardiograph," *Am. Heart J.*, **39**:161, 1950.)

illustrates the circuit diagram of the ballistocardiograph which consists principally of a group of strain gages arranged as a Wheatstone bridge, so that vertical impacts upon the steel platform produce a strain which unbalances the bridge. Sample traces are shown in Figure 21.

### Torsional Ballistocardiogram

The torsional ballistocardiogram can be recorded by using the principle of the torsion pendulum as described by Ernsthausen, vonWit-

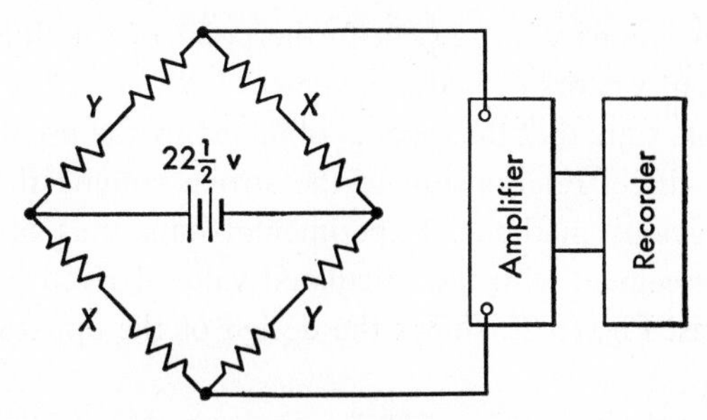


FIGURE 20B. The circuit diagram used in Krahl's electric-strain-gage ballistocardiogram. *X* gages are placed above the recording bar, while *Y* gages are placed beneath it. The signal resulting from an unbalancing of the bridge is amplified and recorded. Placement of the gages above and below recording bar serves to increase the imbalance of the bridge; the two groups (*X* and *Y*) are deformed equally but in opposite directions. The Offner ink-writing oscillograph was used in this instance. (Krahl, V. E.: "The Electric Strain Gauge Ballistocardiograph," *Am. Heart J.*, **39**:161, 1950.)

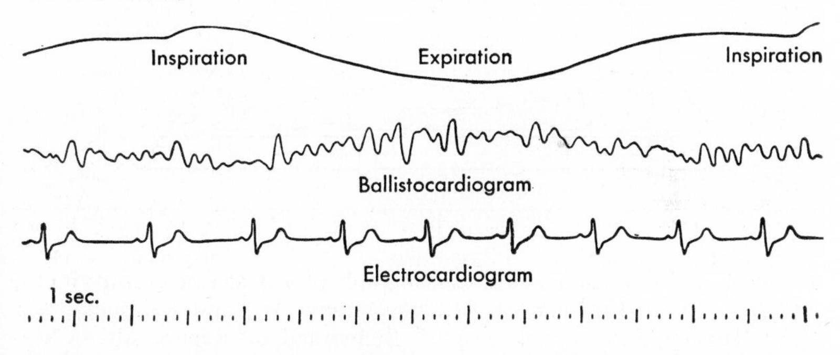


FIGURE 21. Traces obtained by the Krahl electric-strain-gage ballistocardiograph. Simultaneous records of respiration, ballistocardiogram, and electrocardiogram of subject E.G., taken during quiet respiration. The beginning of each respiratory phase is indicated by the word "inspiration" or "expiration." The undulation of the ballistocardiogram's base line, related to the respiratory phases, disappears when the breath is held. Record is about one third actual size. (Krahl, V. E.: "The Electric Strain Gauge Ballistocardiograph," *Am. Heart J.*, **39**:161, 1950.)

tern, and Reismann (*8*). This method records the movements of a horizontal table suspended so that it may rotate in response to the forces set up by each heartbeat. The subject's body may be placed in different positions with respect to the point of rotation, thus picking up different vectors of body movement.

The authors state that the records obtained by the use of this device bear a more direct relationship to the stroke volume than that provided by previous methods. Experimental data thus obtained were in general agreement with the calculated value derived by theoretical considerations. Figure 22 shows the design of the apparatus, Figures

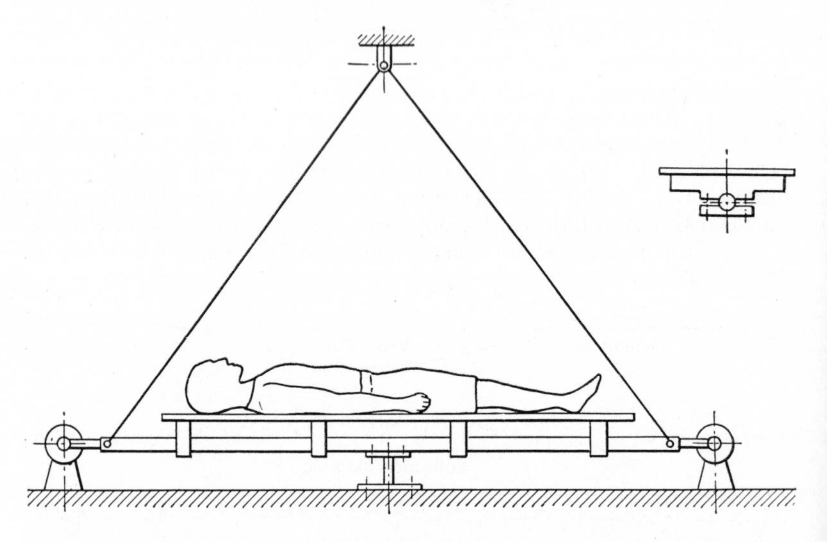

FIGURE 22. The torsion ballistocardiograph of Ernsthausen, vonWittern, and Reismann. (Ernsthausen, W., vonWittern, W., and Reismann, K.: "The Torsion Ballistocardiograph," Memorandum Report MCREXD-696-116A, 29 June 1948. U.S. Air Force, Air Material Command, Wright Patterson Air Force Base, Dayton, Ohio.)

23A and 23B show two possible positions of the subject, and Figure 24 shows a drawing of traces taken with subjects in "middle" and "transverse" positions.

## Tilting Ballistocardiograph

In 1943, Wilkins (*9*) described a tilting ballistocardiograph with which he was able to take traces in the horizontal, upright, and head-down positions. His apparatus is shown in Figure 25, and sample traces are given in Figure 26.

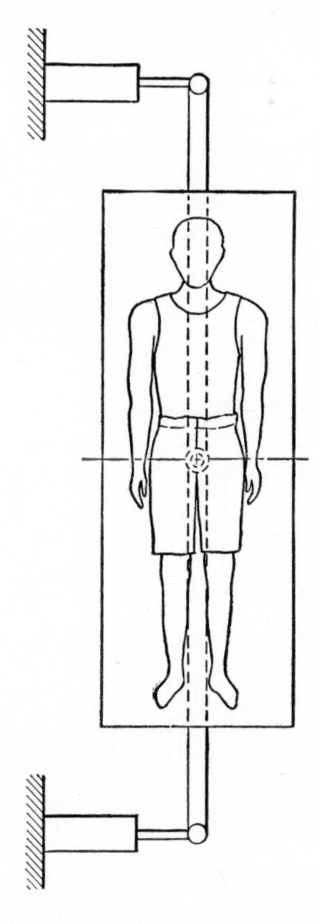

FIGURE 23A. Subject lying on torsional ballistocardiograph table in longitudinal position. (Ernsthausen, W., vonWittern, W., and Reismann, K.: "The Torsion Ballistocardiograph," Memorandum Report MCREXD-696-116A, 29 June 1948. U.S. Air Force, Air Material Command, Wright Patterson Air Force Base, Dayton, Ohio.)

**Direct-body Ballistocardiographs**

Recently Dock and Taubman described three methods for recording movements directly from the body (*10*). The first, after Hamilton (*11*), uses a glycerin-filled capsule held against the head, as shown in Figure 27. The pressure changes in the fluid system produced by body motion were recorded by a standard Cambridge Simplitrol device (Figure 28).

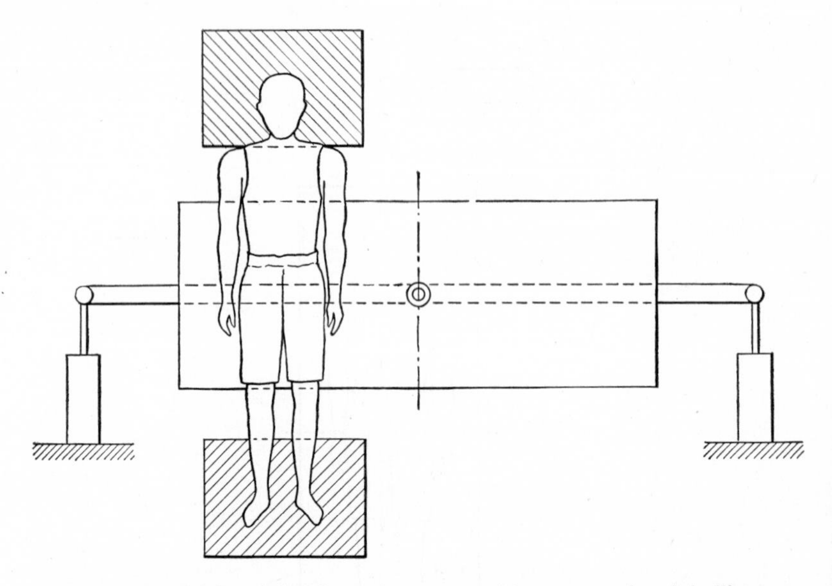

FIGURE 23B. Subject lying in transverse position on torsional ballistocardiograph table. (Ernsthausen, W., vonWittern, W., and Reismann, K.: "The Torsion Ballistocardiograph," Memorandum Report MCREXD-696-116A, 29 June 1948. U.S. Air Force, Air Material Command, Wright Patterson Air Force Base, Dayton, Ohio.)

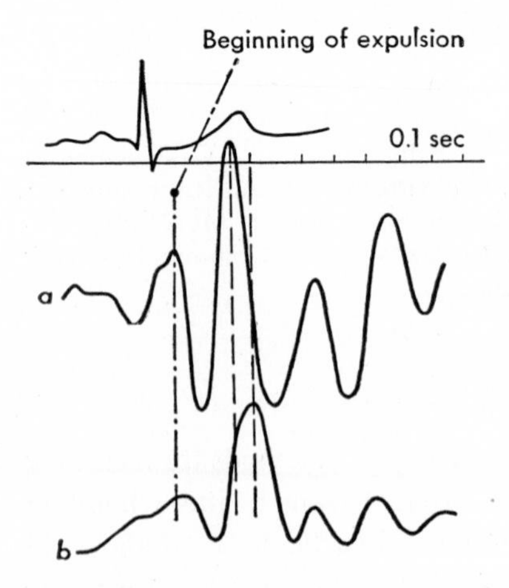


FIGURE 24. Drawing of traces from torsional ballistocardiograph using middle (*A*) and transverse (*B*) positions with simultaneous electrocardiogram at the top. (Ernsthausen, W., vonWittern, W., and Reismann, K.: "The Torsion Ballistocardiograph," Memorandum Report MCREXD-696-116A, 29 June 1948. U.S. Air Force, Air Material Command, Wright Patterson Air Force Base, Dayton, Ohio.)

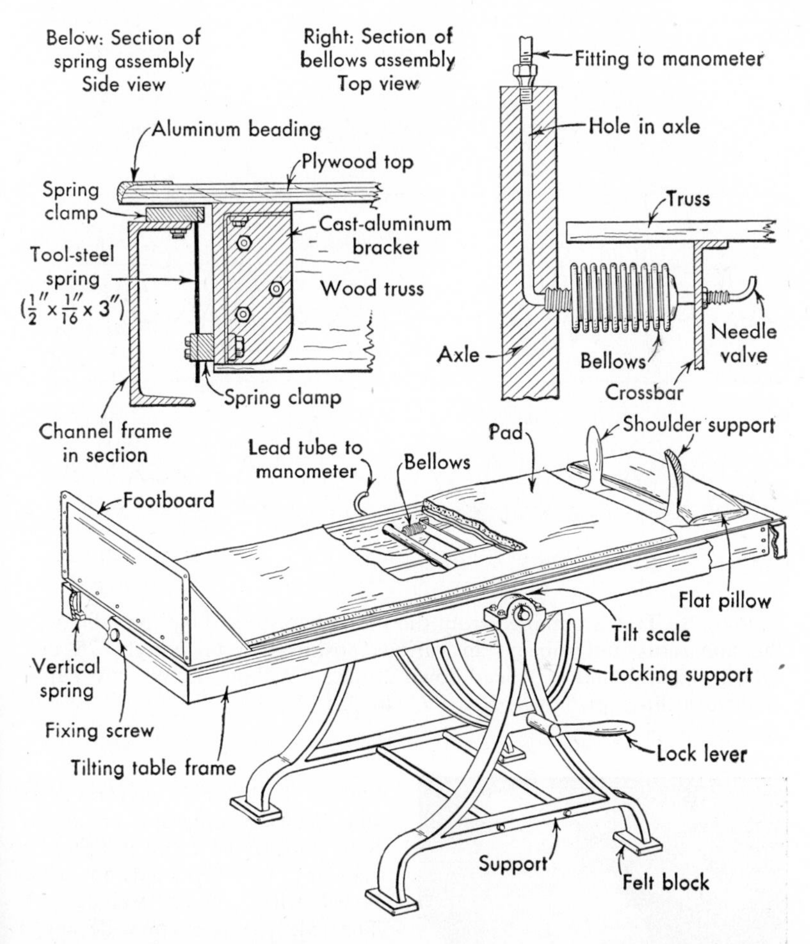


FIGURE 25. The tilting ballistocardiograph table as designed by Wilkins. When the tilting table was set in any desired position, indicated by a graduated scale attached to the frame at the end of the axle, it could be rigidly clamped in that position by screwing tight the lock lever at the side of the frame. Then the fixing screw at the end of the frame was released to allow the ballistocardiograph bed to move. The side cock on the Hamilton manometer was closed, and the apparatus was ready to record the motions of the ballistocardiograph imparted to the bellows and, thence, to the Hamilton manometer. (Wilkins, R. W.: "A Tilting Ballistocardiograph," *Am. Heart J.*, **26**:351, 1943.)

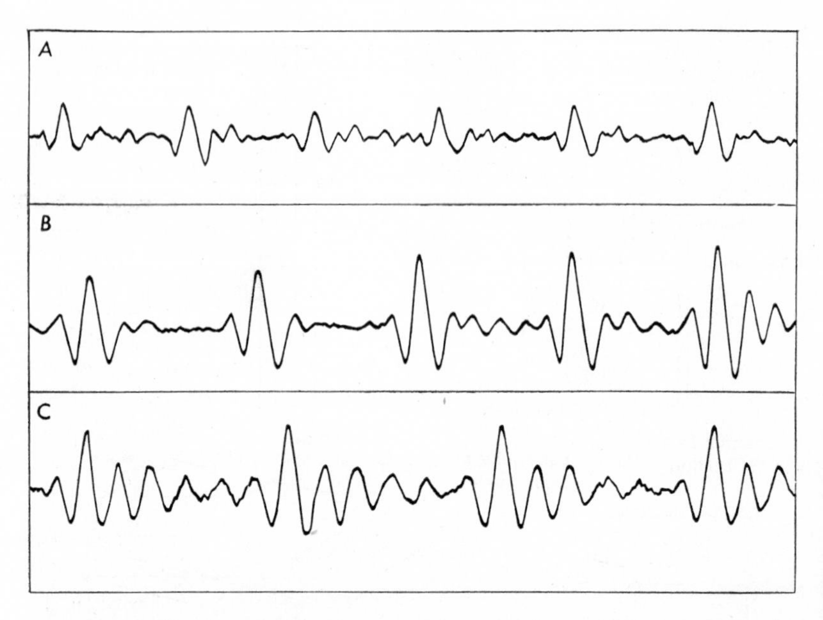


FIGURE 26. Traces obtained from the tilting ballistocardiograph table with the apparatus and subjects in various positions: (*A*) upright 75 deg, (*B*) horizontal, and (*C*) head down 20 deg. (Wilkins, R. W.: "A Tilting Ballistocardiograph," *Am. Heart J.*, **26**:351, 1943.)

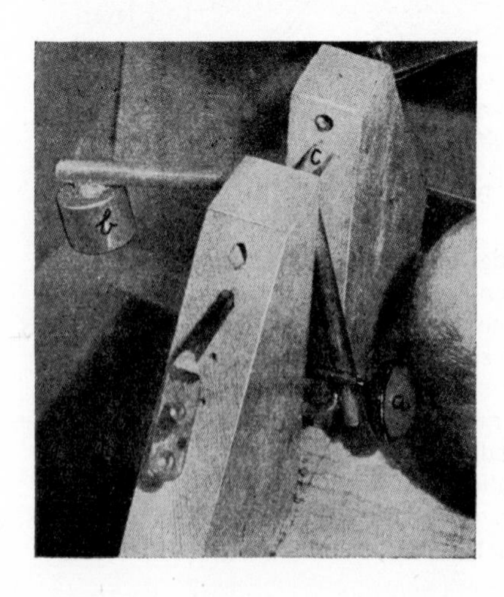


FIGURE 27. Dock's glycerin capsule ballistocardiograph apparatus. Sphygmographic receiver (glycerin capsule) (*a*) mounted on headboard with counter weight (*b*). The axle (*c*) is 6 cm wide and 1 cm in diameter; the counterweight is 400 gm. The axle may be set either 22 or 23.5 cm from the baseboard; the receiver and counterweight are centered 15 cm from the axle. (Dock, W., and Taubman, F.: "Some Techniques for Recording the Ballistocardiogram Directly from the Body," *Am. J. Med.*, **7**:751, 1949.)

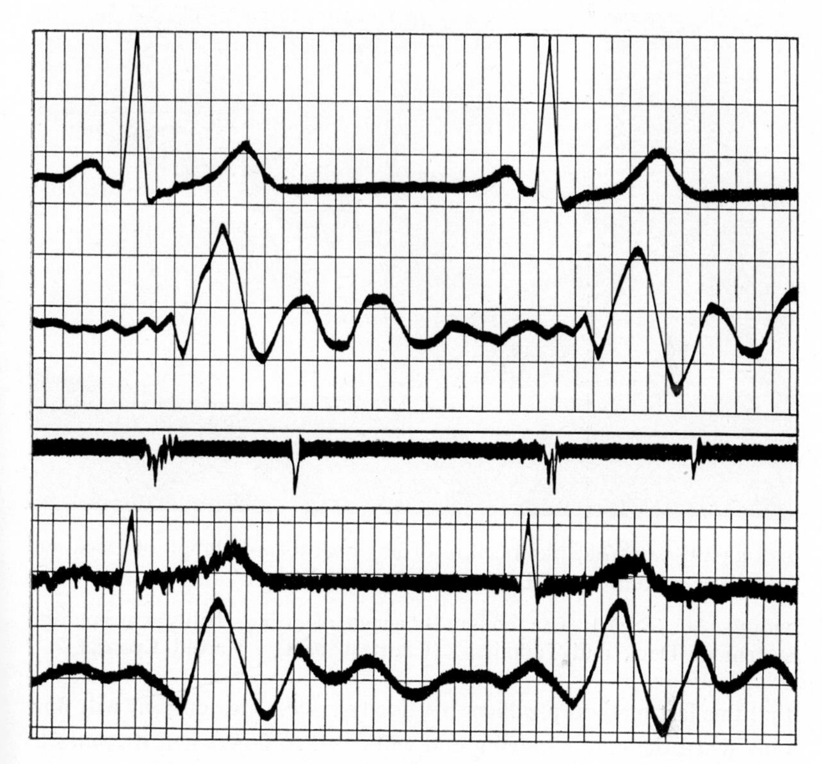

FIGURE 28. Dock's Simplitrol records obtained from the capsule recording system of Figure 27. (Dock, W., and Taubman, F.: "Some Techniques for Recording the Ballistocardiogram Directly from the Body," *Am. J. Med.*, **7**:751, 1949.)

In the second, a light source and photoelectric cell are set up so that the amount of light hitting the photoelectric cell is increased or decreased by movements of the body back and forth. This is accomplished by attaching a piece of cardboard firmly to either the head or the shins, so that its edge partially occludes the light source (Figure 29).

The third method utilizes a coil and permanent-magnet arrangement so that as the body moves, the coil moves with it (in this case the coil is attached to the shins), thereby cutting the lines of force of the magnet and generating a current (Figure 30). It is to be noted

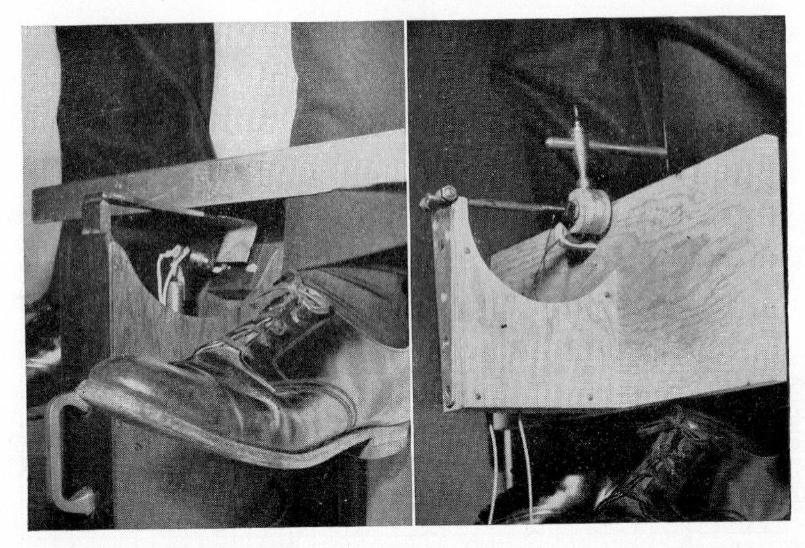

FIGURE 29 *(Left).* The photocell recording ballistocardiograph of Dock and Taubman. (Courtesy of Dr. Harold Lyons.)

FIGURE 30 *(Right).* The coil-and-magnet recording ballistocardiograph system of Dock and Taubman. (Courtesy of Dr. Harold Lyons.)

that this last method produces a velocity trace, since current will flow only when the coil is moving and will cease to flow when it comes to rest. Figure 31 compares traces taken from the shins by the photoelectric and electromagnetic methods (velocity and displacement traces).

### *The Sanborn Ballistocardiograph*

The Sanborn ballistocardiograph (Figure 32) was developed commercially utilizing Dock's photoelectric cell apparatus. This instrument utilizes the principle of placing the transducer element on the shins of a patient riding on his dorsal pads, without the use of a suspended table. Instead of an electromagnetic transducer, as in the Dock system, there is a photoelectric arrangement which is designed to give a frequency response that is flat in the lower regions, as in the case of the Nickerson table, but the upper frequencies are registered even beyond those of the Starr table.

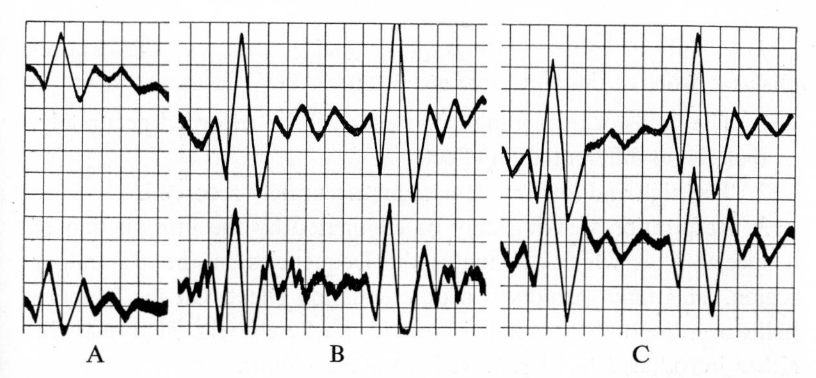


FIGURE 31. Traces taken with Dock and Taubman's apparatus. Electromagnetic trace (lower) and photocell trace (upper), simultaneous record from the shins. Note that changes in velocity (electromagnetic trace) occur 0.02 to 0.06 second before change in position becomes apparent in records *A* and *B* made without a low-pass filter, while the peaks and troughs are practically synchronous in record *C* inscribed with the filter, in this case 100 microfarads across the leads. (Dock, W., and Taubman, F.: "Some Techniques for Recording the Ballistocardiograph Directly from the Body," *Am. J. Med.,* **7**:751, 1949.)

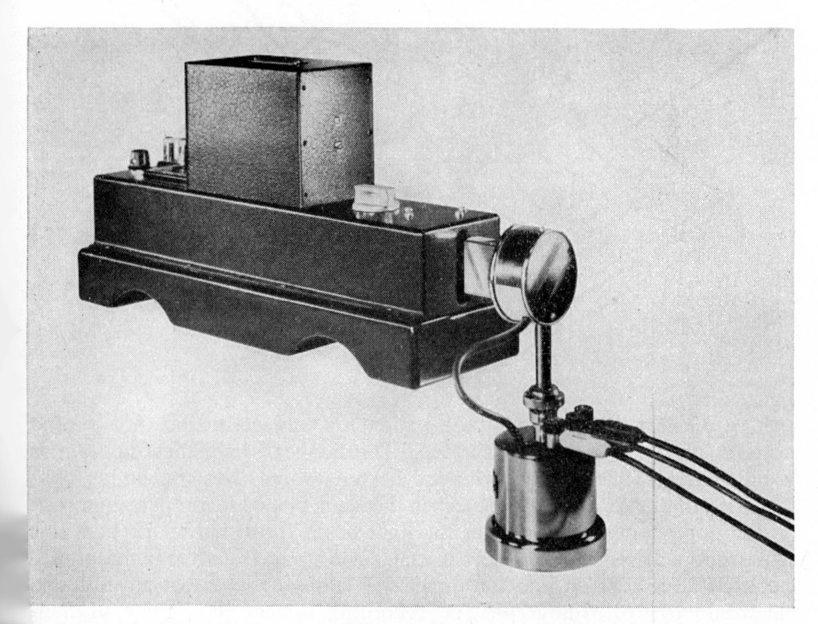

FIGURE 32. The Sanborn ballistocardiograph, a photoelectric type of recording system. (Courtesy of Sanborn Instrument Co., Cambridge.)

The Sanborn ballistocardiograph engineers state that the over-al characteristics of the apparatus are that:

1. The ballistocardiographic K-waves will be recorded accurately as there is no differentiation effect.

2. The high and low frequencies are accurately recorded.

3. Respiration weaving may be eliminated by the introduction o a special filter which attenuates the frequencies in the respiratory region. This filter introduces a differentiation effect. On the Sanborn ballistocardiograph a switch is provided whereby the filter may be either introduced to or removed from the circuit.

The patient or subject lies in a supine position on a hard-surface table (Figure 33). The head may rest on a pillow. The heels are raised

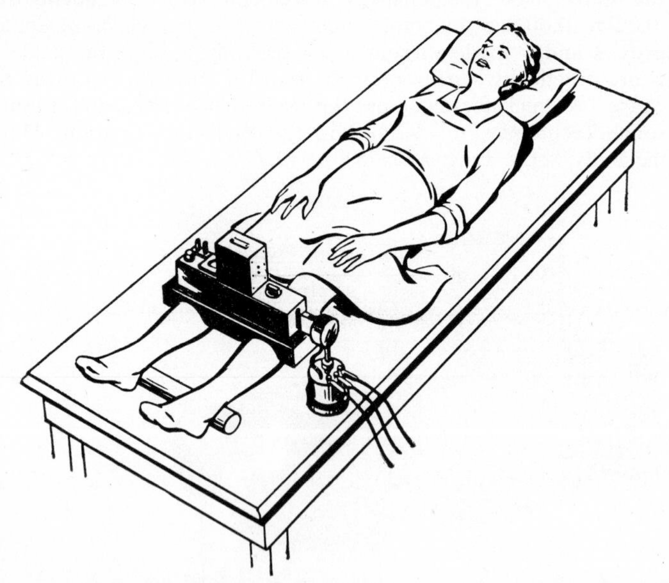

FIGURE 33. An illustration of the patient or subject resting in a supine position on a table or hard surface. The Sanborn ballistocardiogram i lying on the patient's shins with the heels elevated thus preventing con tact with the table. The photoelectric device is placed in proper alignmen on the nonmoving table, so that the light beam from within the box uni will swing across the photoelectric cell. The three leads from the photo electric device pass on into the three limb leads for lead I of any suitable electronic electrocardiograph-type recording system. (Courtesy of San born Instrument Co., Cambridge.)

from contact with the table by a suitable support. The body then rests on its dorsal pads when the ballistic circulatory thrusts are imparted to it.

The substantial boxlike frame rests on the patient's shins, and as it rides with each axial movement of the body, a sharply defined light beam of standard intensity swings across the window of a photoelectric device placed in proper alignment on the nonmoving table or surface. The light beam is created by a power source within the unit.

The moving field of light regulates the stationary photoelectric cell proportionately to the ballistic thrusts, and the three limb lead wires of an electronic-type recorder are connected to the photoelectric system. It is recommended that the electrocardiogram be turned to lead I position and that sensitivity be adjusted for optimum deflection of the electrocardiogram. A sensitivity of 1 centimeter/1 millivolt deflection is not necessarily used. For standardization purposes a 1-millivolt signal may be used for comparisons over a period of time.

### *The Glennite Ballistocardiograph*

The new Glennite ballistocardiograph (Figures 34 and 35), made by the John Peck Laboratories of New York, is a simple system which operates on a piezoelectric crystal type of pickup. The firm and heavy base with the Glennite unit rests on the nonmoving hard surface or bed, and the heavy steel bar is placed across the patient's shins. The resulting trace is one of a displacement type.

Figure 36 is a normal trace obtained with the Glennite ballistocardiograph.

Figure 37 shows simultaneous records of heart sounds, Glennite ballistocardiogram, and electrocardiogram obtained with this unit. The record is abnormal as to both pattern and type; there is also an abnormally increased respiratory variation of the complexes.

## General Discussion of Types of Ballistocardiographs

These attempts to simplify the means of recording the ballistocardiogram are ingenious, and certainly they point the way to future

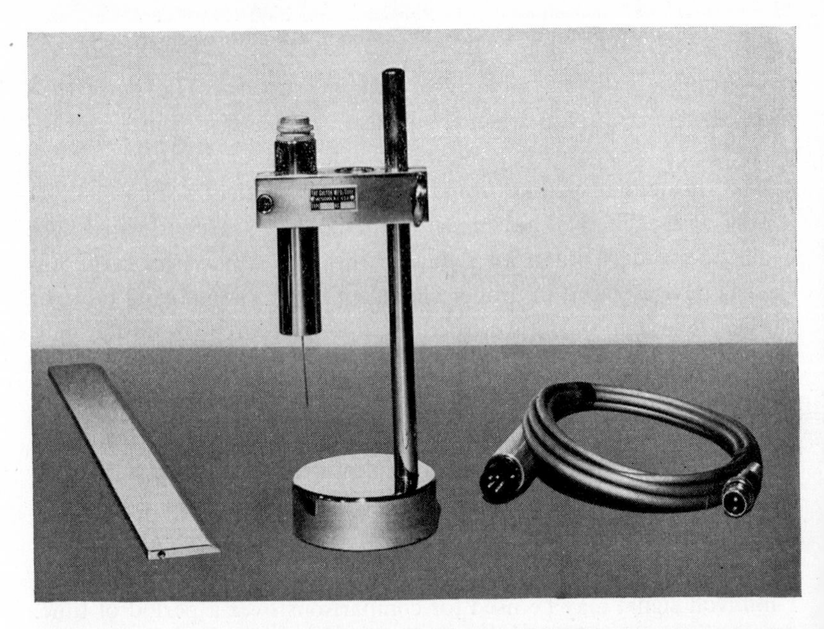

FIGURE 34. The complete Glennite ballistocardiograph apparatus consisting of (from the left) a steel shin bar which is properly placed contiguous with the movable arm attached to the Glennite unit (Glennite system), which may be adjusted upward or downward, and the wire and plug adapted to any electronic-type direct-writing electrocardiograph. (Courtesy of John Peck Laboratories, Inc., New York, N. Y.)

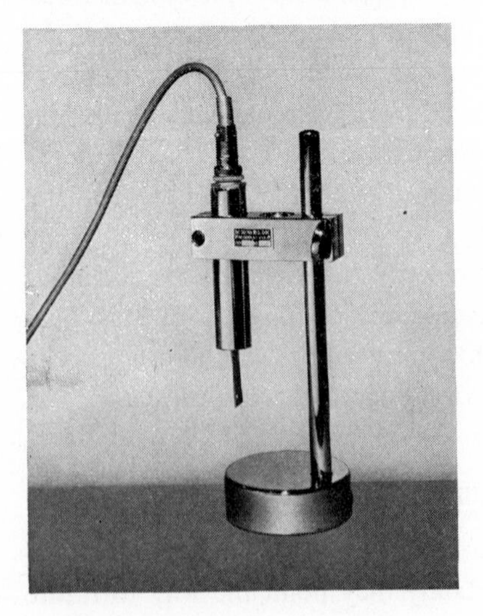

FIGURE 35. A close-up of the Glennite unit showing system plugged in ready for operation. (Courtesy of John Peck Laboratories, Inc. New York, N. Y.)

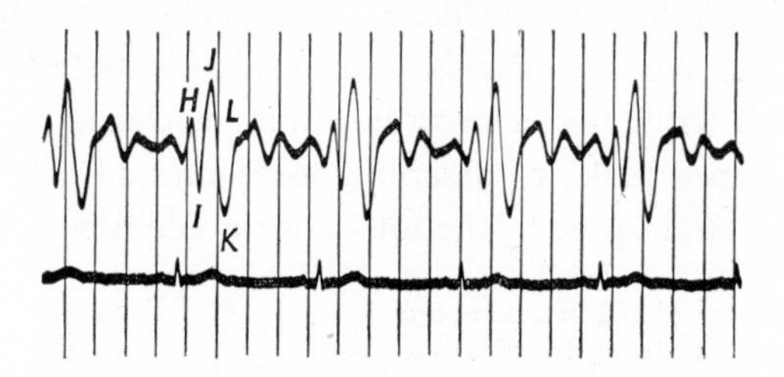


FIGURE 36. A normal trace obtained with the Glennite ballistocardiograph. (Courtesy of John Peck Laboratories, Inc., New York, N. Y.)

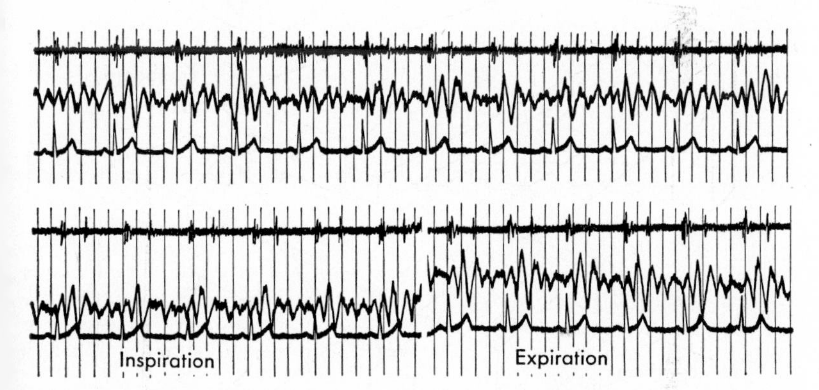


FIGURE 37. The middle trace in each instance shows the ballistocardiograph obtained by this Glennite unit. The record is abnormal in pattern and type and shows an increased degree of respiratory variation of the complexes. (Courtesy of John Peck Laboratories, Inc., New York, N. Y.)

clinical use. However, because of present difficulties with body movements and reproducibility of patterns, it is our opinion that a table offers the best immediate clinical means, to date, of recording the ballistocardiogram. Three types of tables are available for clinical work: vertical, torsional, and horizontal. There is no doubt that the vertical and torsional tables will be properly utilized after basic clinical studies have been completed. The choice of the horizontal table at present depends upon the fact that the extensive studies of normal subjects and clinical material thus far reported have utilized this medium. This does not preclude the possibility that future investigation will reveal other methods to be of greater clinical value.

For those interested in immediate clinical ballistocardiography, an easy method has recently become available. This system utilizes an ordinary direct-writing electrocardiograph machine, a "high-frequency" undamped table, as described in Figures 11 and 12, and a Statham piston strain gage.* The total cost in addition to that of the

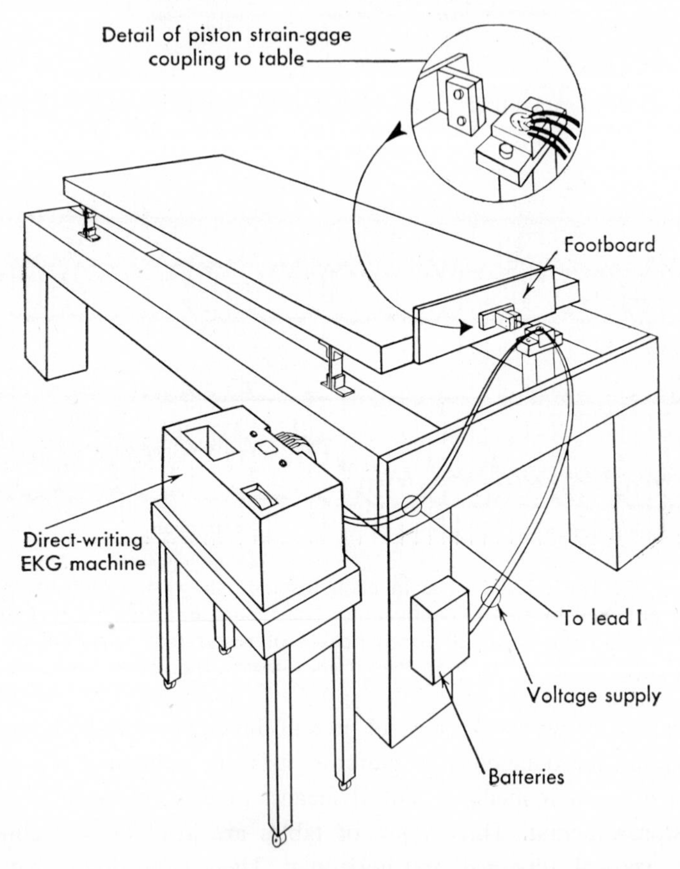


FIGURE 38. The high-frequency ballistocardiograph table adapted for routine recordings through a direct-writing electrocardiograph apparatus.

electrocardiograph machine is estimated at not more than $200. The mounting for the gage and the connections to the electrocardiograph machine (via any lead) can be seen in Figures 38 and 39. The output

* Statham Laboratories, Inc., Beverly Hills, Calif.

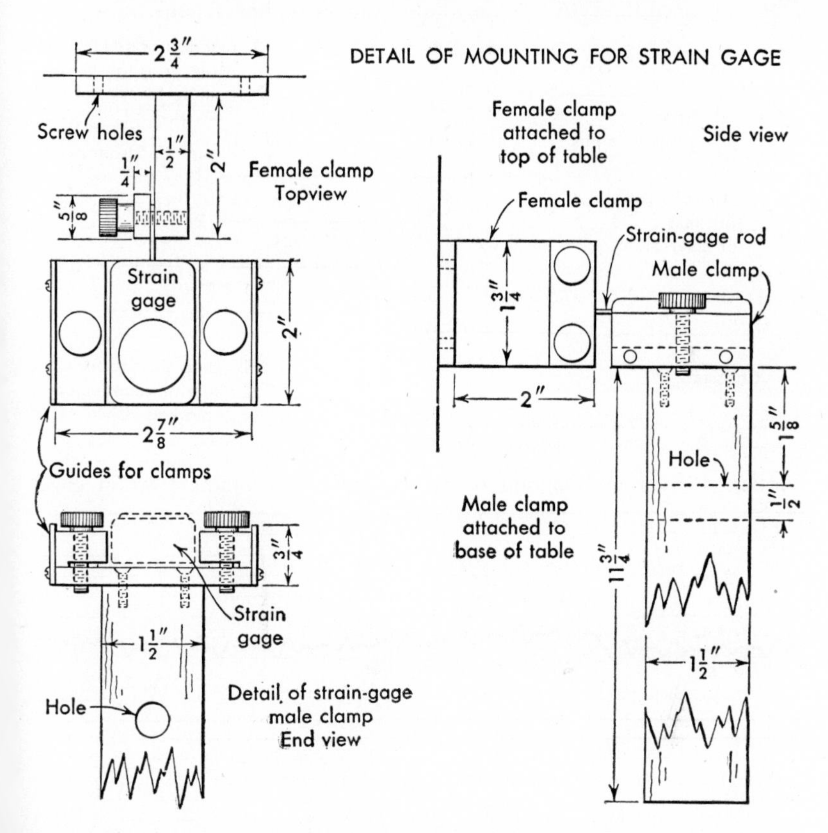


FIGURE 39. Details of mounting for the Statham strain gage on the high-frequency table shown in Figure 38.

of the gage will vary with the voltage applied (from a dry-cell battery), the maximum possible voltage being 25 volts. A wide range of amplitude of records can be obtained if the gage is supplied with 24 to 25 volts. The desired voltage can be obtained from a 45-volt battery. A variable series resistance and a voltmeter are placed in the circuit so that any voltage up to 25 volts can be accurately applied to the gage. See Figure 40 for details of the circuit diagram of this control unit.

Standardization of the ballistocardiogram with this apparatus can be accomplished either by adding a known force to one end of the

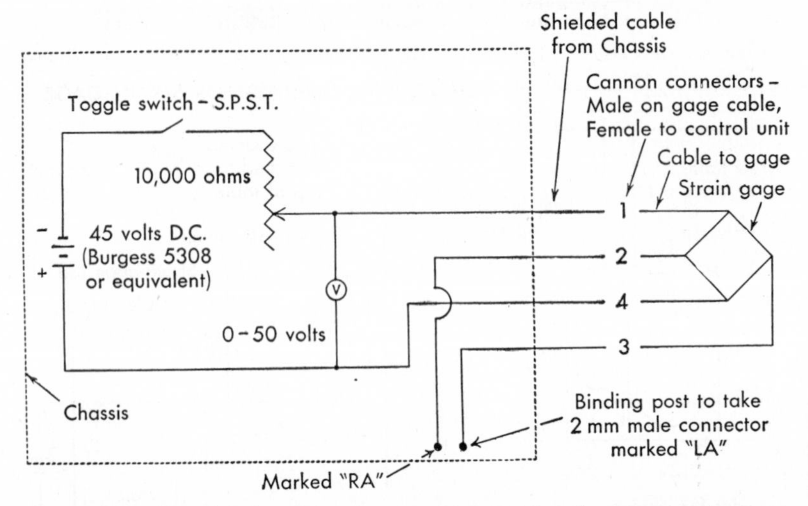


FIGURE 40. Circuit diagram of power supply for Statham strain gage.

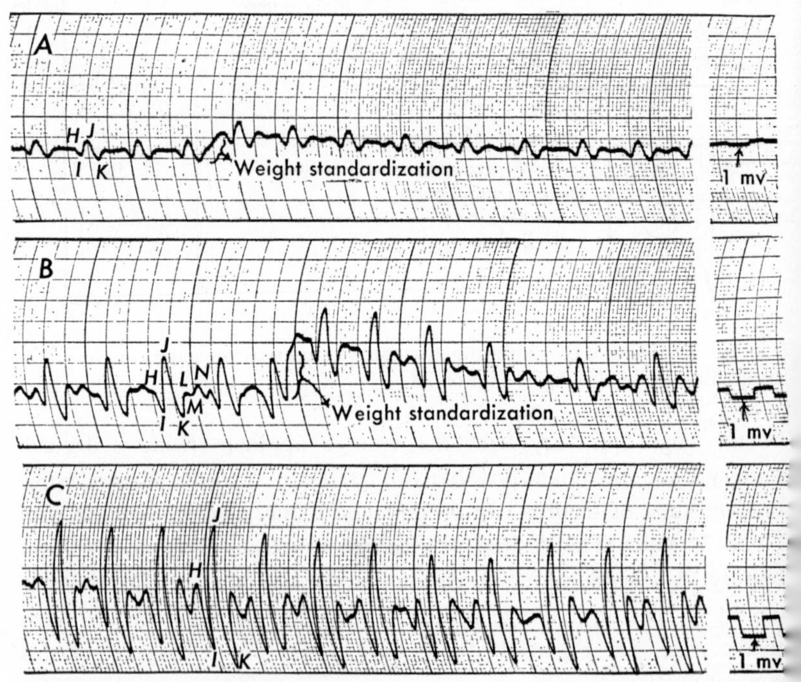


FIGURE 41. Normal ballistocardiogram records obtained from a direct-writing Eden electrocardiograph. Both weight and electrical standardization are shown in traces *A* and *B*.

table (as described elsewhere) or by maintaining the gage voltage constant at 24 or 25 volts and applying a standard millivolt stimulus through the electrocardiograph machine (Figure 41). The height of the millivolt deflection can be used in evaluating the amplitude of the IJ stroke, after a suitable number of normals have been observed by this method.

## REFERENCES

### APPARATUS


1. Starr, I., Rawson, A. J., Schroeder, H. A., and Joseph, N. R.: "Studies on the Estimation of Cardiac Output in Man, and of Abnormalities in Cardiac Function, from the Heart's Recoil and the Blood's Impacts; the Ballistocardiogram," *Am. J. Physiol.,* **127**:1, 1939.
2. Blair, H. A.: Personal communication.
3. Brown, D. E.: "The Design of the Ballistocardiograph," *J. Clin. Investigation,* **21**:294, 1942.
4. Nickerson, J. L., Warren, J. W., and Brannon, E. S.: "The Cardiac Output in Man; Studies with the Low Frequency, Critically-damped Ballistocardiograph, and the Method of Right Atrial Catheterization," *J. Clin. Investigation,* **26**:1, 1947.
5. Starr, I., and Rawson, A. J.: "The Vertical Ballistocardiograph: Experiments on the Changes in the Circulation on Arising: with a Further Study of Ballistic Theory," *Am. J. Physiol.,* **134**:403, 1941.
6. Krahl, V. E.: "A Simple Laboratory Apparatus for Demonstration of Cardiac Ballistics," *Science,* **105**:393, 1947.
7. Krahl, V. E.: "The Electric Strain Gauge Ballistocardiograph," *Am. Heart J.,* **39**:161, 1950.
8. Ernsthausen, W., vonWittern, W., and Reismann, K.: "The Torsion Ballistocardiograph," Memorandum Report MCREXD-696-116A, 29 June 1948. U.S. Air Force, Air Material Command, Wright Patterson Air Force Base, Dayton, Ohio.
9. Wilkins, R. W.: "A Tilting Ballistocardiograph," *Am. Heart J.,* **26**:351, 1943.
10. Dock, W., and Taubman, F.: "Some Techniques for Recording the Ballistocardiogram Directly from the Body," *Am. J. Med.,* **7**:751, 1949.
11. Hamilton, W. F., Remington, J. W., and Dow, P.: "Relationship between Cardiac Ejection Curve and Ballistocardiographic Forces," *Am. J. Physiol.,* **144**:557, 1945.

CHAPTER THREE

# Physical Considerations in the Construction of a Ballistocardiograph

Edgar D. Seymour—Arthur W. Tyler, Ph.D.—Miller R. Hutchison
*Development Department*
*Eastman Kodak Company*
*Rochester, New York*

---

FIGURE 42 shows a simple mechanical system made up of a mass coupled to ground through a spring and subjected to an oscillating force from some driving system. If the ratio of the frequency of the driving force to the natural frequency of the mass and spring is small compared to unity, then a record of the displacement of the mass will be proportional to the force exerted by the driving system. If, however, this ratio is large, compared to unity, the record will be proportional to the displacement of the driving system. If this ratio is near unity the system will be driven by a frequency near its own natural frequency, and the trace will be distorted in amplitude and phase; such a trace will be neither a force trace nor a displacement trace. If there is controlled damping in this simple system, the amplitude distortion near unity frequency ratio can be reduced. However, phase distortion still occurs (*1*).

Critical damping is defined as that amount of damping which will just prevent the oscillation of the mass when it has been drawn away from its neutral position and released. Seven tenths of this critical damping is considered the best compromise, as this gives minimum distortion of amplitude and a linear phase shift as the frequency ratio

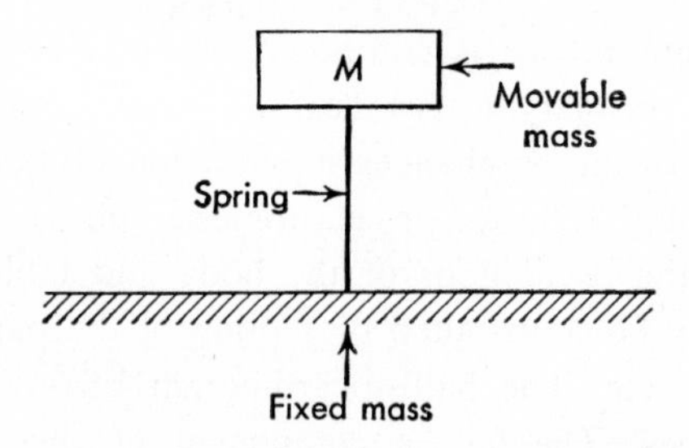


FIGURE 42. A drawing of a simple mass and spring arrangement (1 deg of freedom). In this system the driving force is applied to the movable mass. If the spring is stiff so that the spring and mass have a high natural tendency with respect to the frequency of the driving force, then the record obtained from the deflections of the movable mass will be a force trace. If the spring is weak, so that the spring and mass have a low natural frequency with respect to the frequency of the driving force, then the record obtained from the deflections of the movable mass will be a displacement trace. If the natural frequency of the spring and mass approximates that of the driving force then the trace obtained will be neither a force nor a displacement record, but will be distorted in amplitude and phase.

approaches unity. A linear phase shift will result in a time delay of recorded signals, but it causes no distortion by unequal relative shifts of different frequency components.

The Starr type of ballistocardiograph table is constructed with very stiff springs, giving it a relatively high natural frequency so that we are measuring the force necessary to hold the patient stationary. A ballistocardiograph table with a human body upon it is not so simple as the system described in the preceding paragraph. It will have several degrees of freedom. The body can be considered as made up of many springs and masses with interdamping. In addition, there are a hydraulic pump (heart) and elastomeric tubes (arteries and veins) which are the sources of the driving forces. These tubes and pump can be considered to be supported in a nearly rigid frame (skeleton) by springs (tissue) with damping. This frame is coupled to the table by other springs (fleshy part of body and clothes) and a footboard. It should be noted that forces occurring simultaneously in opposite directions within the body will to some extent cancel one another. The record shows only the net unbalanced longitudinal forces with respect to time. The complete ballistocardiogram record is composed of the algebraic sum of all forces: i.e., the primary forces (cardiac and respiratory), the hydraulic forces (owing to changes in direction of fluid and pressure waves moving and reflected in elastomeric tubes), and the forces resulting from the oscillations of the body and table and whatever background may be contributed by motion of the patient, movement of the building, etc. The ballistocardiogram record is made up of many frequencies. The largest component of these frequencies is about 5 or 6 cycles per second. This is approximately the natural frequency of a warm cadaver on the ballistocardiograph table. The prominence of this frequency indicates that the body is caused to oscillate at its own natural frequency by the forces which we are endeavoring to measure. The damping within the body is such that these oscillations die out fairly rapidly (approximately 1 cardiac cycle). Considerable caution should be exercised in the interpretation of the ballistocardiogram record, since the presence of the relatively large oscillation at the body's natural frequency masks that portion of the record which is due to the primary forces. In addition to a relatively small direct record, the primary forces also cause an augmentation or suppression of the body oscillation, depending on the phase with which they occur.

In addition to the relatively low natural frequency (5 to 6 cycles) attributable to the body, there should also be another natural frequency as determined by the ballistocardiograph table-top springs and the mass of the table and body. This frequency will not be the same as that obtained when an equivalent dead weight replaces the body, because of the flexibility of the body. The fact that this frequency does not appear in the traces obtained with a warm cadaver on ar undamped table indicates that the damping contributed by the bod is considerable, and the addition of further damping on the ballisto cardiograph table itself will not alter the results appreciably. Further more, the use of critical damping for the purpose of measuring strok volumes is unnecessary since the formula used to compute strok volume from the IJ stroke amplitude contains an arbitrary constar which is empirically derived and can be changed at will.

A low-frequency ballistocardiograph table is constructed with wea springs, giving it a relatively long period. It permits the patient move relatively freely in space. Consequently, the record is one of body displacement—not of force. It has been noted that these records are generally similar to the records obtained with a high-frequency table. This similarity is due to the predominant sinusoidal body-frequency component which has the same shape in both records.

The interesting portion of the record in both cases consists of the small irregularities directly due to the primary causes, and the resulting change in amplitude of the body oscillations. These features of the records are different in the two cases.

It should be pointed out that the type of equipment used to pick up the table displacement also will determine the type of record obtained. If an instrument which measures displacement (such as a strain gage) is used, then the table displacement is recorded as such. If a coil-and-magnet arrangement, such as a magnetic loud-speaker, is used to pick up the table movements, then the record is a velocity trace of the table displacement.

It appears from the foregoing that it is advantageous to use a relatively high-frequency undamped table. The reasons for this can be summarized briefly: (1) Since, ultimately, it is the actual forces in the body with which we are concerned, rather than table displacement, it is reasonable to use a high-frequency table which gives a force trace directly. (2) If it becomes desirable to know the rate of change of the forces involved, it will be necessary to differentiate the high-frequency ballistocardiogram trace only once with respect to time, whereas, if a low-frequency table is used, the displacement record obtained must be differentiated three times with respect to time.* † (3) The bulk of the clinical and experimental work to date

* Let $s$ be the position of the low-frequency table; then the curve obtained will be $s = f(t)$. The second differential of this with respect to time will be $\left(\frac{d^2s}{dt^2}\right) \sim F$ where $F$ is equal to the force that causes the body and table to move. To obtain the rate of change of this force it is necessary to differentiate this equation with respect to time again $\frac{(d^3s)}{(dt^3)} \sim \frac{(dF)}{(dt)}$. With the high-frequency table, $F$ is measured directly, and the rate of change of $F$ can be obtained by differentiating this curve with respect to time $\frac{dF}{dt}$.

† The pattern of rate of change of force may be useful, for instance, in understanding the circulatory dynamics that occur in aortic insufficiency, where the records obtained with our present device (force traces) are frequently within the normal limits, and where high amplitude of IJ stroke occurs. A differentiation of this trace may enable us properly to evaluate the abnormality.

has been done with a high-frequency table. (4) The traces obtained from a low-frequency table are different from those obtained from a high-frequency table, and this complicates their interpretation in terms of the accumulated data.

With this in mind, certain desirable characteristics of the high-frequency ballistocardiograph table can be listed:

1. The table-top springs should be stiff to keep the natural frequency high.
2. The table top should be light in weight for the same reason.
3. The table top and base should be rigid, to reduce artefacts.
4. The footboard should be rigid, and good coupling of the patient to the footboard should be obtained. In this respect, possibly a device similar to a dentist chair's headrest could be used to hold the patient against the footboard.
5. The base of the table should be very heavy. This will allow the table top to oscillate with minimal interference from the movements of the building.
6. The base should be isolated from its support to minimize the effects of building vibrations, as by using ball-bearing steel wheels fixed to roll only in head-to-foot direction upon a thick steel plate.
7. The pickup should be located to minimize distortions due to flexures of the table top.
8. There should be no cushions between the patient and table top.

## REFERENCES

### THE PHYSICS OF BALLISTOCARDIOGRAPH CONSTRUCTION

1. Freberg, C. R., and Kemler, E. N.: *Elements of Mechanical Vibration,* John Wiley & Sons, Inc., New York, 1943, p. 56, Fig. 3–11.

CHAPTER FOUR

# The Normal Ballistocardiogram

IN the previous chapters we have discussed the historical background of ballistocardiography and described methods by which the ballistocardiogram can be obtained. The usefulness of these records is related to the fact that normal heart patterns have the same characteristics and are reproducible. The following description of the normal ballistocardiogram is concerned only with records of body forces made on a relatively high-frequency, undamped table. These were obtained almost entirely with a capacitance transducer (*1*), but any force records using a similar table will be comparable.

## Characteristics of the Normal Ballistocardiogram

The ballistocardiogram complex is the pattern of movements of the table with each heartbeat. A single complex is shown in Figure 43A. Upward deflections are movements of the table toward the head, and downward deflections represent footward movements of the table. The pattern begins with a small headward deflection that starts its rise during the QRS complex of the electrocardiogram. This wave has been called the H-wave by Starr, and the subsequent movements are the I-J-K-L-M-N-O waves. Ordinarily, each beat is described as being made up of two groups of waves—the H-I-J-K waves making up its main body, and being followed by the so-called "after waves," L-M-N-O.

The ballistocardiogram may be described as to the regularity and

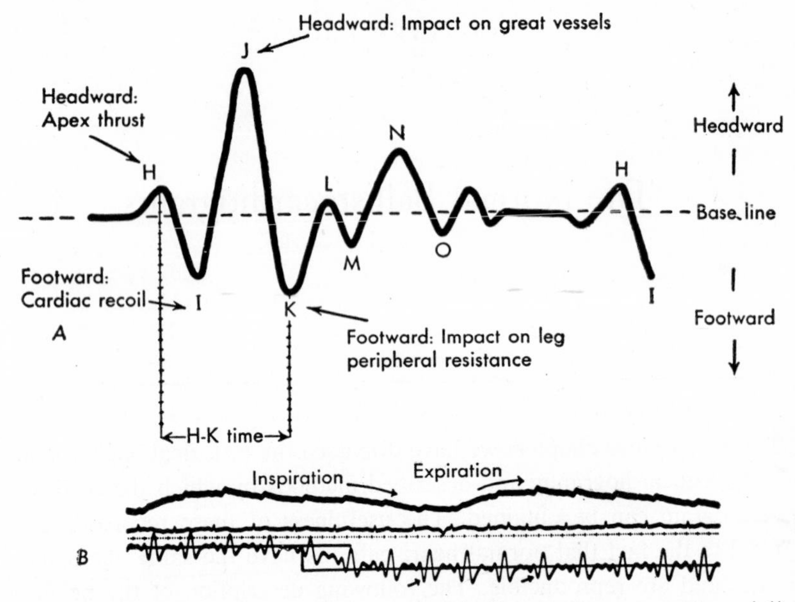


FIGURE 43. Drawing of a single normal ballistocardiogram pattern (*A*) and reproduction of a normal trace (*B*). (Modified from Brown, H. R., Jr., and deLalla, V., Jr.: "The Ballistocardiogram, Description and Clinical Use," *Am. J. Med.*, **9**:718, 1950.)

definitiveness of each beat pattern, the "absolute" amplitude of the pattern, the relative amplitude of the component waves, the variations with respiration, and the constancy of the H-K time; in the future, other temporal relations may be found to be of value. Figure 43B shows normal adult ballistocardiograms. In this record, as in most of the figures, there are four channels presented. They are: (1) respiration—top undulating line, inspiration represented by a downward deflection and expiration by an upward deflection; (2) electrocardiogram—ordinarily this is lead II; (3) ballistocardiogram—a downward shift in the base line seen in most of the records is the weight standardization which is due to a 285-gm force applied to the table in a footward direction; (4) time lines, with 0.04 sec between the smaller marks, and 0.2 sec between the large ones. These tracings demonstrate the various characteristics of the normal ballistocardiogram.

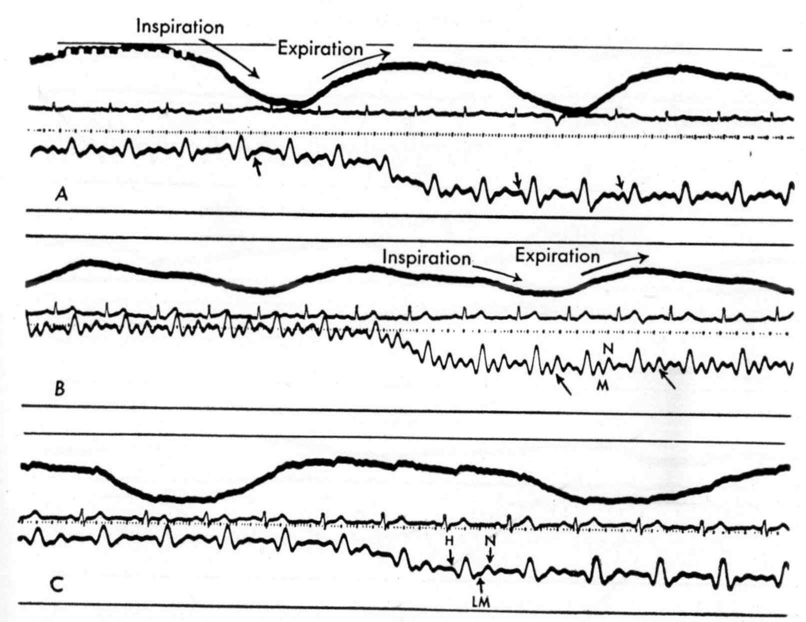


FIGURE 44. Three normal ballistocardiograms in adults. (*A*) First arrow shows flat LM stroke; note the following N peak. Second arrow shows decreased to flat H peak in inspiratory phase. Third arrow shows increased H peak in expiratory phase. (*B*) Note the inspiratory increase of the MN stroke (arrow). (*C*) Arrows point to flat H-wave and flat LM stroke. Note the very definite N peak following the flat LM stroke. (Modified from Brown, H. R., Jr., and deLalla, V., Jr.: "The Ballistocardiogram, Description and Clinical Use," *Am. J. Med.,* **9**:718, 1950.)

The regularity of the beat pattern is important, because the pattern is irregular in serious cardiac pathology. The normal pattern is unchanging in appearance from beat to beat except for slight variations of amplitude with respiration (Figures 44 and 45).

The onset of each normal complete pattern is definite, although when the rate is rapid the H-wave may be obscured by oscillations from the previous beat. In any case, the normal HI stroke is always obvious (Figures 44 and 45).

Our third consideration of the normal ballistocardiogram is the amplitude of the waves. Ordinarily, we judge the amplitude of a pattern by the length of the IJ stroke, since this has been closely

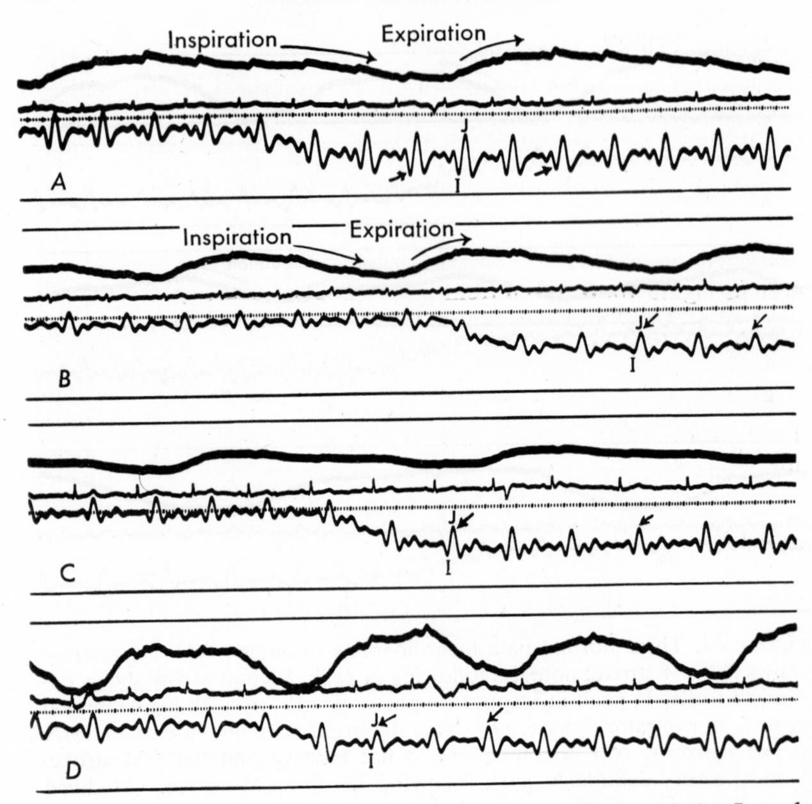


FIGURE 45. Note respiratory variations in the amplitude of the I- and J-waves (arrows). The records are all normal ballistocardiograms.

related to the output of the heart. A rough estimate of adequacy of amplitude is the relation of IJ to the weight standardization. Normally, the IJ stroke is equal to at least one half the distance the base line moves with the application of the weight, and usually it is greater than that. The IJ amplitude varies slightly with respiration, and it will be seen in Figure 45 that the IJ strokes during inspiration are larger than those in expiration. Normally, the difference is small, and the record becomes abnormal when the "respiratory variation" increases. A quantitative estimate of cardiac output and the degree of respiratory variation can be made (Chapter 5).

A fourth important normal characteristic is the constancy of the

H-K time. This is measured from the peak of the H-wave to the deepest part of the K-wave. It varies from one person to the next, but it is constant in any individual to within 0.01 sec (*2*). It seems reasonable that H-K time might vary with the height of the subject since it is proportional to the time interval between the onset of cardiac ejection and the arrival of the impulse wave in the legs (see H- and K-wave analysis). This has been found to be the case, as will be seen in Figure 46, *B,* taken from Brown and deLalla (*2*). This shows a fairly good direct relationship between the height and the H-K time. H-K time does not vary with cycle length (Figure 46, *A*). The H-K interval is normally constant and has been found to vary in certain pathological states, such as congestive failure and congenital heart disease (*2*).

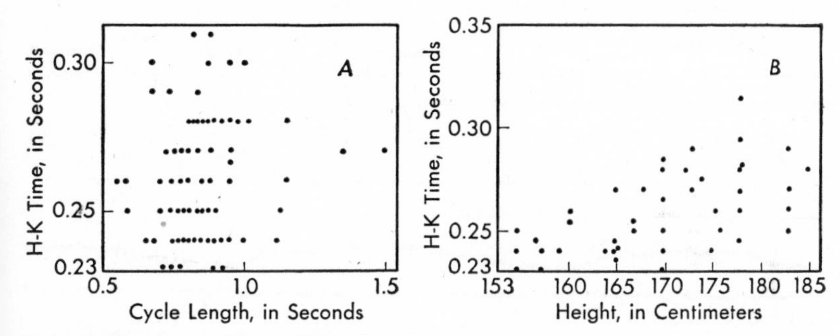


FIGURE 46. (*A*) Graph of H-K time (measured in seconds between the H peak and the K valley) against cycle length in seconds (measured from the J peak of the preceding beat to the J peak of the beat in question). Note the absence of relationship. (*B*) Graph of H-K time against height of subject in centimeters. Note the tendency of the H-K time to increase with height. (Brown, H. R., Jr., and deLalla, V., Jr.: "The Ballistocardiogram, Description and Clinical Use," *Am. J. Med.,* **9**:718, 1950.)

Each individual stroke comprising the single beat pattern must be studied in its relation to others. For this purpose a base line can be used. In general the after waves of the preceding beat present a useful means of determining where the base line should be drawn. If the rate is slow, there will be no difficulty, since the after waves will be reduced to a straight line (Figure 47, *A*). In more rapid rates the base line can be drawn with considerable accuracy by observing the oscillations which follow the N peak and determining where the base line would have been if there were no succeeding beat (Figure 47, *B*).

*H-wave*

The variation of the H-wave from normal to normal is perhaps greater than any other component of the pattern. It may be low or flat (Figure 47, *A*), or it may be relatively high (Figure 45). Ordinarily, the H peak is approximately one fourth the size of the J peak,

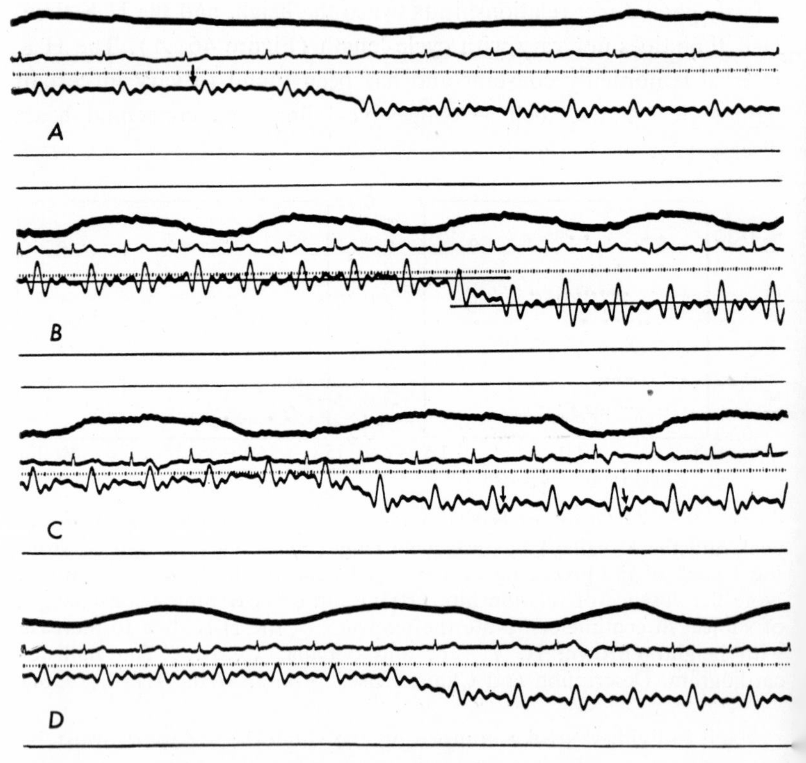


FIGURE 47. Four normal ballistocardiograms in adults. (*A*) Slow rate with easily identified base line. Note flat H-waves. (*B*) More rapid rate with base line drawn in accordance to method in test. The standardization would be measured as the distance between the two lines. (*C*) Note the respiratory variation of the LM stroke (arrows). (*D*) Shows very little respiratory variation. (Brown, H. R., Jr., and deLalla, V., Jr.: "The Ballistocardiogram, Description and Clinical Use," *Am. J. Med.*, **9**:718, 1950.)

and less than the I valley. It has been suggested by Hamilton (*3*) that this first upward deflection is initiated by the apex thrust which occurs during isometric contraction. Figure 48 shows the simultaneous relations of the onset of the H-wave to the apex thrust, and to the first heart sound and to mechanical auricular systole. It can be seen that the onset of the H-wave is simultaneous with the apex thrust and the first heart sound.

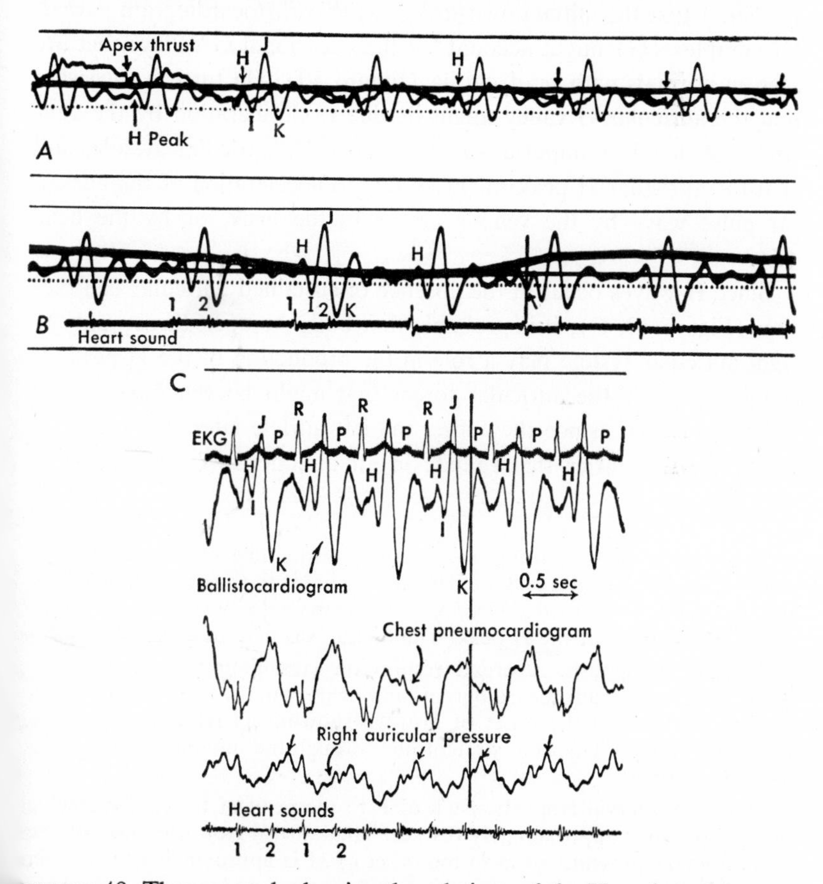


FIGURE 48. Three records showing the relations of the H peak to the apex thrust (*A*), heart sounds (*B*) and (*C*), and mechanical auricular systole.*

(*A*) Simultaneously recorded respiration (solid heavy black line), ballistocardiogram, and apex thrust. The apex thrust was recorded through

*(Caption continued on next page)*

Nickerson suggested a second mechanism for the production of the H peak (*4*). He observed a ballistic pattern following auricular systole in complete heart block. We have confirmed this observation (Figure 49, *A* and *B*). It is evident that the time interval between electrical auricular systole (EKG P-wave), and the auricular ballistocardiogram H-wave in heart block is of the same magnitude as the normal P-H interval (0.2 to 0.3 sec). It was suggested by one of us (V.deL.) that the initial downstroke of the ballistocardiogram auricular complex (G) might account for the occasional G valleys that are seen in normals with bradycardia (Figure 50). He further suggested that the auricular G valley might be due to deceleration by the ventricles of blood or impulse wave generated by auricular systole, and that the auricular H peak might be due to deceleration of the auricular pulse wave by the venous arches in the neck, or by the head (5).

Since H-waves occur in the absence of sustained auricular contraction (Figure 49, *C*), it is probable that both the apex thrust and the right auricular systole play a role in the production of the H peak. It is fair to ignore the auricular forces that might be generated in the pulmonary veins, since they enter the left auricle laterally, and since they have tributaries that radiate in all directions. Therefore, these

---

a piezoelectric crystal, using an inverted thistle tube over the point of maximal impulse as the pickup. The arrows point to the onset of the apex thrust (sharp downward deflection). Note the relationship of the apex thrust to the onset of the H peak. The breath was held in expiration.

(*B*) Simultaneously recorded respiration (undulating heavy line, inspiration down), ballistocardiogram, and heart sounds. Arrow points to a line drawn through the onset of H-wave showing its relationship to the first heart sound. The solid straight line through the middle of the tracing has no meaning.

(*C*) The interval from the peak of P to the peak of the first auricular pressure wave is approximately 0.1 sec. The interval from the peak of the first auricular pressure wave to the onset of H is approximately 0.15 sec.

* Record *C* is obtained from the laboratory of Dr. R. Bruce *et al.*, Department of Medicine, University of Rochester School of Medicine and Dentistry, Rochester, N. Y. Auricular pressure was obtained through a cardiac catheter with a Hathaway transducer.

(deLalla, V., Jr., Epstein, M. A., and Brown, H. R., Jr.: "Analysis of H-Wave," *Circulation,* **2**:765, 1950.)

forces would probably cancel out as far as the ballistocardiogram is concerned.

*I-wave*

In the normals observed thus far, the I valley has always been less than the J peak, and usually greater than the H peak. It varies in size

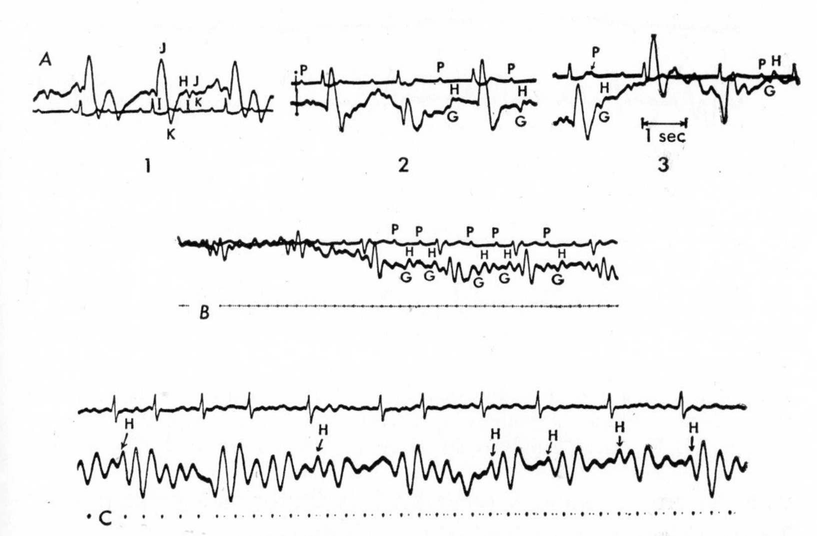


FIGURE 49. Traces *A* (sublabeled 1, 2, 3) are taken from Nickerson. They are from a patient with complete heart block. The lettering in tracing 1 is Nickerson's; all subsequent lettering is ours. Note that Nickerson's I valley corresponds to our G valley and that his J peak corresponds to our H peak. The small peak that Nickerson has labeled H is probably an artefact since it does not repeat. These small ballistic complexes represent auricular systole and demonstrate the relationship of auricular systole to the H-wave. Note the P-H and P-G intervals.

Tracings *B* and *C* are from our files. *B* is from a patient with complete heart block and shows the auricular ballistic complex (G valley and H peak). Note the P-G and P-H intervals.

Tracing *C* is from a patient with auricular fibrillation. Note the presence of H peaks, although there is no sustained auricular mechanical systole. This is taken to mean that the apex thrust also plays a role in producing the H peak.

(Traces *A* from Nickerson, J. L.: "Some Observations on the Ballistocardiographic Pattern, with Special Reference to the H and K Waves," *J. Clin. Investigation,* **28**:369, 1949. Traces *B* and *C* from deLalla, V., Jr., Epstein, M. A., and Brown, H. R., Jr.: "Analysis of H-Wave," *Circulation,* **2**:765, 1950.)

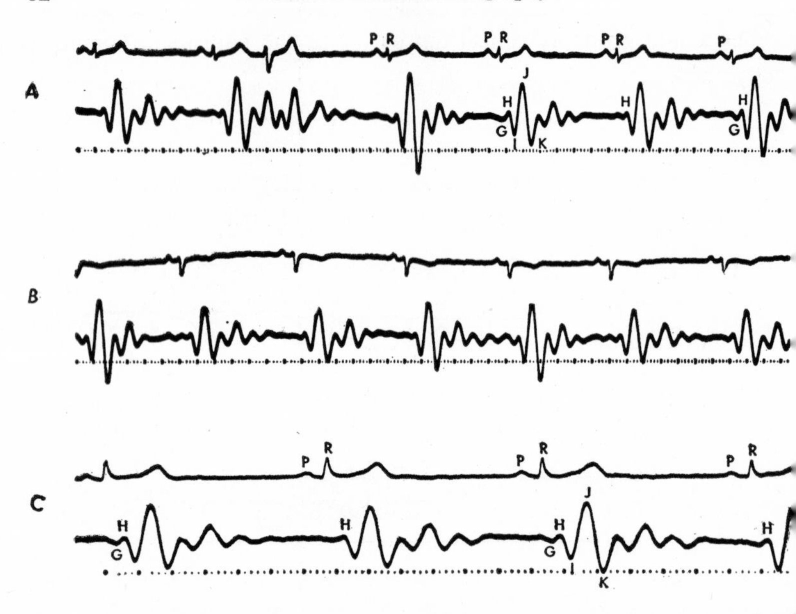


FIGURE 50. Relations of electrocardiogram P-wave to G valley and H peak. Note definite G valleys. (deLalla, V., Jr., Epstein, M. A., and Brown, H. R., Jr.: "Analysis of H-Wave," *Circulation,* **2**:765, 1950.)

with different individuals; generally, it is approximately one half the J peak (Figures 44, 45, and 47).

The downward I-wave may be caused by the footward component of the cardiac recoil accompanying ventricular ejection (*3* and *6*). It can be seen from Figure 48 that the HI stroke occurs at the proper time for this to be true. Possible further evidence for this premise is offered below under the discussion of the respiratory variation of the ballistocardiogram (Chapter 6).

*J-wave*

The J-wave may be due to deceleration of either blood or impulse wave or both, by the aortic and pulmonic arches, and possibly by the head. Originally, the J peak was thought to be caused by the impact of blood on the arch of the aorta (*6*). Recent and continuing work in our laboratory has suggested that this may not be the case. The kinetic energy required is too great, and it seems more reasonable that a pulse wave or "bulge" of the great vessels, traveling at relatively high speed, is responsible for the J-wave. The force of the deceleration of this impulse in the pulmonary arches, aorta, and neck vessels would be great.

Starr's original use of the ballistocardiogram was based on the premise that the height of the IJ stroke is directly proportional to the stroke volume of the heart. The earlier theories about these waves ignored the pulmonary circulation, but certain of our observations suggest that impacts in the pulmonary circulation play an important part in producing the ballistocardiogram. The respiratory variation of the IJ stroke in normal and abnormal subjects is in the same direction as the respiratory variation of both the right heart stroke volume and the total stroke volume; this is good confirmation of the theory that the IJ stroke is caused by forces set up by both right and left ventricular systole. Also, we have observed Diodrast angiocardiograms, made with the cinefluorograph (*8*), that demonstrate large pulmonary arteries with strikingly vigorous systolic impacts, in both normal and abnormal individuals. These findings lead to the conclusion that the lesser circulation cannot be ignored, though direct proof of the part it plays is not yet available.

The theory that the IJ stroke is related to the cardiac output is not invalidated by the premise that the IJ stroke is caused by deceleration of a pulse wave rather than blood flow, for it seems probable that the magnitude of the pulse-wave bulge is proportional to the stroke volume. However, in certain cases sclerotic vessel walls might lead to erroneous results.

The IJ stroke is the highest normal upward deflection, and it may be regarded as a means of estimating the stroke volume and the forcefulness of cardiac ejection (Figures 44, 45, and 47). In normals and abnormals where the pattern is regular enough, it is possible to arrive at figures for the stroke and minute volumes (in cubic centimeters) by Starr's method (*6* and *7*) (see Chapter 5).

However, it is not routinely necessary to compute the cardiac output by such measurements, for one can arrive at gross and practical estimates by comparing the IJ stroke with the standardization. The standardization is accomplished by allowing a 280-gm weight to exert a constant pull upon one end of the table. The resulting shift in the base line is then proportional to the sensitivity of the apparatus and is useful in computing or estimating the cardiac output. The ratio of the IJ stroke to the standardization is constant for any individual at a given time, regardless of the sensitivity (Figure 51).

In a series of 100 normals, using this method of standardization, we have observed that the ratio of the IJ stroke to the standardization is usually more than ½ (Figures 44, 45, and 47). In large subjects it may be 1 or more (Figure 51); in small individuals it occasionally is slightly less than ½. With this simple method it is possible to approximate cardiac outputs in general terms of low, normal, or high. It must be stated, however, that each newly constructed ballistocardio-

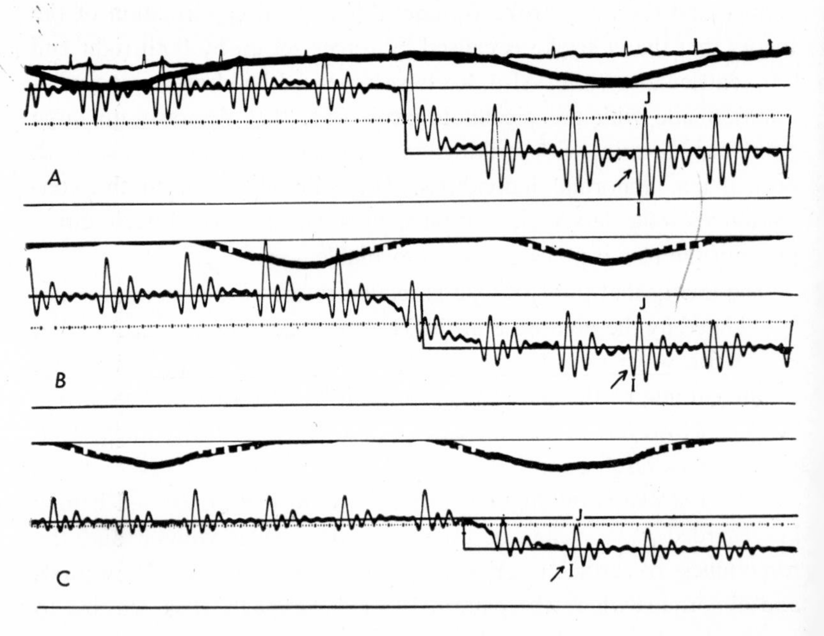


FIGURE 51. Three tracings on a large man showing the effects of varying sensitivity. Note that although the IJ stroke and the standardization (distance between base lines) increase with increased sensitivity (highest in *A*, least in *C*), the ratio of the IJ stroke to the standardization is constant. The standardization is measured as the shift of the base line produced by the addition of a constant weight to one end of the ballistocardiograph table. (See text for description.) The base lines are drawn in.

graph will have its own sensitivity characteristics and must be standardized in this respect.

*K-wave*

This wave is a sharp footward deflection coming directly after the J peak. Normally, the IJ and JK strokes are almost mirror images of each other (Figures 44, 45, and 47). Frequently, in normal subjects the K-waves are slightly deeper than the I-waves, particularly in expiration. The JK stroke probably represents the deceleration of the footward impulse wave by the arteriolar peripheral resistance in the legs (*3*). There is a considerable amount of evidence to support this. In hypertension, where the peripheral resistance is increased, the K-wave is deepened and usually returns to normal when the blood pressure is lowered by sympathectomy or by veratrum viride (Figure 52).



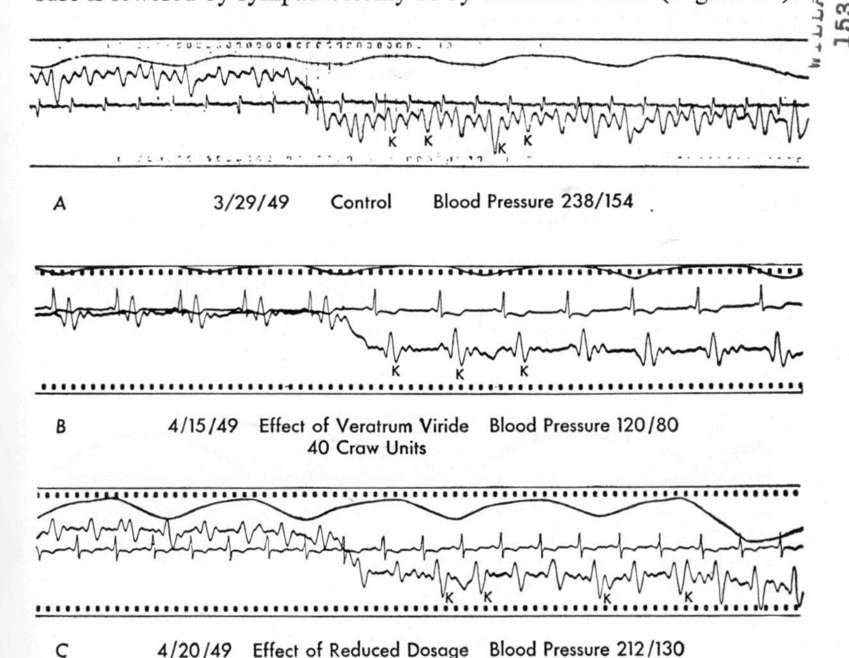


FIGURE 52. Tracings *A*, *B*, and *C* are on the same hypertensive subject. Note the deep K-waves in *A* (control). When the tension is lowered by veratrum viride the K-waves become normal (*B*).

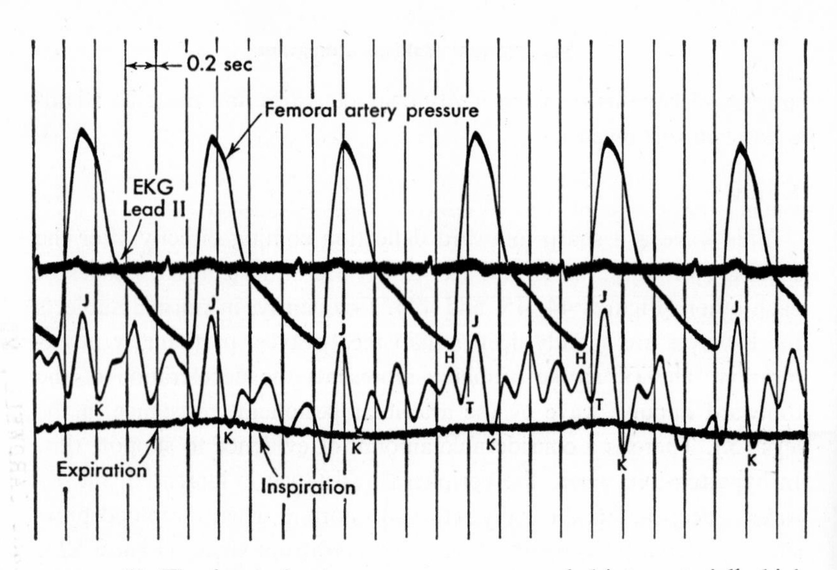


FIGURE 53. The femoral artery pressure was recorded intra-arterially high in the groin. The time it would take for the peak pressure wave to reach smaller leg arterioles probably accounts for the short interval between peak femoral pressure and onset of JK stroke.

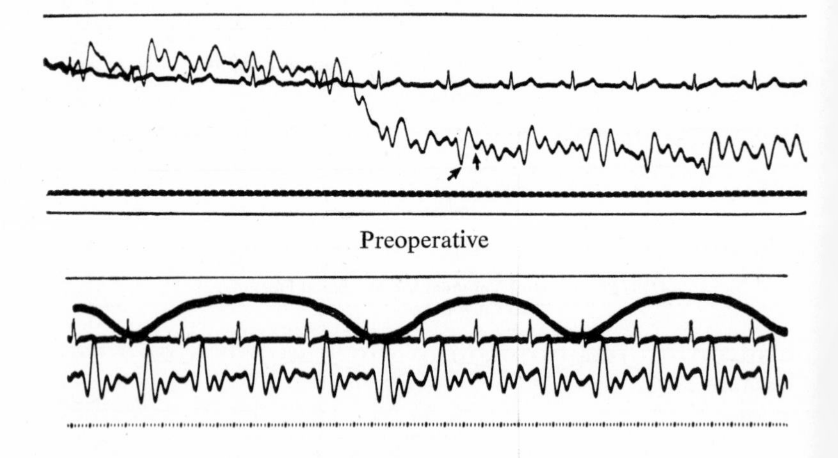


FIGURE 54. Coarctation of the aorta before and after operation. (Brown, H. R., Jr., Hoffman, M. J., and deLalla, V., Jr.: "Ballistocardiograms in Coarctation of the Aorta," *New England J. Med.,* **240**:715, 1949.)

Note the relationship of the JK stroke to the peak pressure in the femoral artery (Figure 53). Nickerson has shown that the length of the aorta probably plays a role in the production of the K-wave by varying the length of a model aorta (*4*). He showed that a shorter aorta produced a shorter K valley in traces obtained from his model. Also, in coarctation of the aorta the K-waves are shallow and return to normal after operation (*3, 9, 10,* and *11*) (Figure 54).

*The After Waves*

The L-M-N-O-waves are known as the "after waves," since they occur after the completion of mechanical cardiac systole. They will be obscured frequently by tachycardia, tachypnea, dyspnea, or phase oscillations. As previously stated, the L- and N-waves are headward, and the M- and O-waves are footward deflections. We do not yet know what forces are responsible for these waves. It is probable, however, that the after waves are not simple oscillations trailing off from the IJK deflections. There are two explanations for this theory. First, the after waves do not gradually fall off in amplitude as their distance from JK becomes greater. As a matter of fact, N-wave follows L, and yet it is usually higher than L. In the second place, we do not think the after waves are simple harmonic vibrations, because they are modified in certain pathological conditions (see Chapter 8).

## REFERENCES

### NORMAL BALLISTOCARDIOGRAPH


1. Brown, H. R., Jr., and Pearson, R.: "A New Electronic Method for Simultaneous Recording of the Ballistocardiograph and Electrocardiograph," *Am. Heart J.,* **35**:756, 1948.
2. Brown, H. R., Jr., and deLalla, V., Jr.: "The Ballistocardiogram, Description and Clinical Use," *Am. J. Med.,* **9**:718, 1950.
3. Hamilton, W. F., Remington, J. W., and Dow, P.: "Relationship between Cardiac Ejection Curve and Ballistocardiographic Forces," *Am. J. Physiol.,* **144**:557, 1945.

4. Nickerson, J. L.: "Some Observations on the Ballistocardiographic Pattern, with Special Reference to the H and K Waves," *J. Clin. Investigation,* **28**:369, 1949.
5. deLalla, V., Jr., Epstein, M. A., and Brown, H. R., Jr.: "Analysis of H-Wave," *Circulation,* **2**:765, 1950.
6. Starr, I., Rawson, A. J., Schroeder, H. A., and Joseph, N. R.: "Studies on the Estimation of Cardiac Output in Man, and of Abnormalities in Cardiac Function, from the Heart's Recoil and the Blood's Impacts; the Ballistocardiogram," *Am. J. Physiol.,* **127**:1, 1939.
7. Starr, I., and Schroeder, H.: "Ballistocardiogram—Normal Standards, Abnormalities Commonly Found in Diseases of Heart and Circulation, and Their Significance," *J. Clin. Investigation,* **19**:437, 1940.
8. Olsan, E. S., Watson, J. S., Weinberg, S., and Ramsey, G. H.: Unpublished data, Department of Radiology, University of Rochester School of Medicine and Dentistry, Rochester, N.Y.
9. Brown, H. R., Jr., Hoffman, M. J., and deLalla, V., Jr.: "Ballistocardiograms in Coarctation of the Aorta," *New England J. Med.,* **240**:715, 1949.
10. Nickerson, J. L., Humphreys, G. H., Deterling, R. A., Fleming, T. C., and Maters, J. A. L.: "Diagnosis of Coarctation of Aorta with the Aid of the Low Frequency, Critically Damped Ballistocardiograph," *Circulation,* **1**:1032, 1950.
11. Murphy, R. A.: "Ballistocardiographic Patterns in Intraluminal Aortic Obstructions," *Am. Heart J.,* **39**:174, 1950.

CHAPTER FIVE

# Cardiac Output

THE modern formulae that have been derived for determination of stroke volume are based upon the assumption that the amplitude of the IJ stroke is proportional to the volume of blood ejected from the ventricles. This is probably true in normals; at least, there is good correlation between determinations made from the ballistocardiogram and those made on the same subjects by either the direct Fick method, or the ethyl iodide method (*1, 2, 3,* and *4*). The possibility that this correlation is a coincidence is remote. It is our present opinion that there is a relationship between the height of the IJ stroke and the stroke volume in normals. This may be indirect in as much as the IJ stroke is probably related to the deceleration of the impulse bulge rather than to actual blood flow. However, the size of the bulge is proportional to the volume of blood ejected.

Using this assumption as a starting point, formulae have been derived, chiefly by empirical means. By measuring the stroke volume with other techniques, a constant may be derived for use in the stroke volume formula, which will then give the result in cubic centimeters per beat, when certain measurements from the ballistocardiogram are also used.

Starr's initial formula $SV = K\sqrt{(31 + 2J)\ AC\ \frac{3}{2}}$ was useful and gave good results (*1*). A definition of terms follows.

K represents the constant described above, and equals **7** when the sensitivity of the recording apparatus is such that a 280-gm force applied to the table will cause a 10-mm deflection on the record. We have derived values for K for other sensitivities, so that we can change the gain of our instrument at will. The formula for this derivation is $K = 1.32/W$, where W is the force in grams necessary to move the table 1 mm and K is the constant to be used in the stroke volume formula.

I is the depth of the I valley in millimeters from the base line, and J is the height of the J peak in millimeters above the base line (Figure 55A).

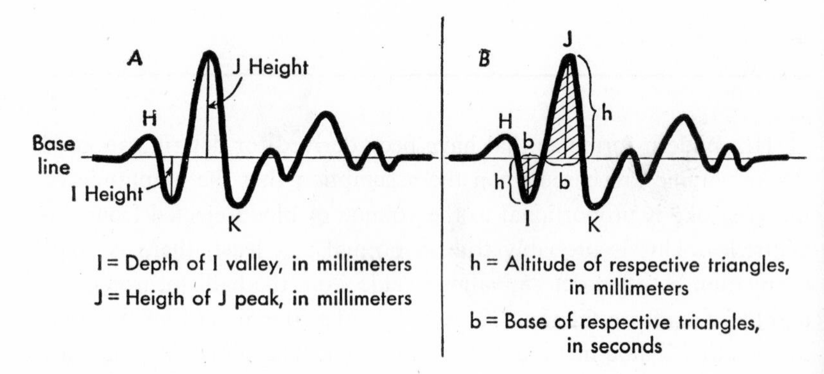


FIGURE 55. (*A*) Technique for measuring I- and J-wave amplitude for the height formula of Starr. (*B*) Technique for obtaining measurements of triangular I and J areas for area formula of Starr.

A represents the cross-sectional area of the aorta in square centimeters, and is derived according to the method described by Bazett (*5*). From the post-mortem data of Suter (*6*), and Dreyer *et al.* (*7*), it is shown that there was a correlation between the cross-sectional area of the aorta and the body surface area. This relationship is shown by the formula $A = (SA \times a) + b$, where a and b are constants derived from the age of the subject and SA is the surface area in square meters. Since b is always a negative number for the internal cross-sectional measurements (Figure 56), Starr rearranged the formula to read: $A = (SA \times a) - b$. Figure 57 shows values for a and b for various ages.

C is the average cycle length in seconds taken from a representa-

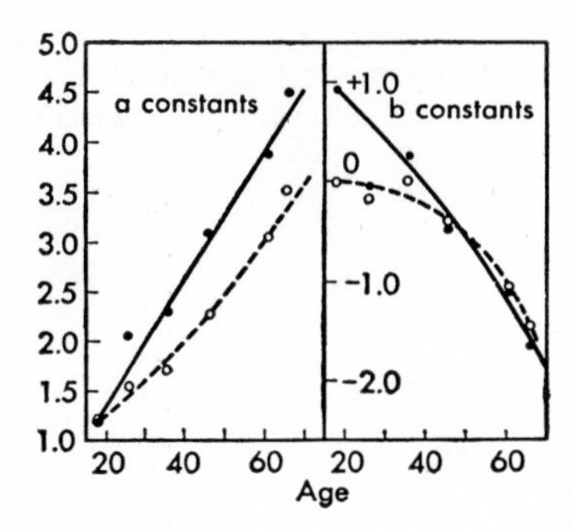


FIGURE 56. Graph showing derivation of a and b constants, after Dreyer *et al.* Constants from which the external and internal cross-sectional area of the ascending aorta may be calculated by the equations given in the text for subjects of different age (abscissae). The heavy lines and solid circles indicate the values for the external cross-sectional area, the dotted lines and open circles those for the internal. (Bazett, H. C., Cotton, F. S., LaPlas, L. B., and Scott, J. B.: "The Calculation of Cardiac Output and Effective Peripheral Resistance from Blood Pressure Measurements with an Appendix on the size of the Aorta in Man," *Am. J. Physiol.,* **113**:312, 1935. Dreyer, G., Ray, W., and Walker, E. W. A.: "The Size of the Aorta in Warm-Blooded Animals and Its Relationship to the Body Weight and to the Surfaces Area Expressed in a Formula," *Proc. Roy. Soc.* (*London*), Series *B,* **86**:39, 1912.)

tive portion of the record. Figure 58 shows C 3/2 values and heart rates for various values of C.

Starr correlated the stroke volume as determined by this formula and the ethyl iodide method in 25 subjects (Figure 59). The coefficient of correlation was 0.86, with a standard deviation of 0.052 (*1*).

Starr (*1*) derived a stroke volume formula using the area under the I- and J-waves: $SV = 33 \sqrt{(2 \text{ area I} + \text{area J}) \text{ AC } 1/2}$, where 33 is the constant necessary to arrive at the stroke volume in cubic centimeters when a 280-gm force causes a 10-mm deflection on the record.

A and C are derived as in the height formula.

The area under I and J is found by creating a triangle for each, where the base of the triangle is the base line, and the altitude is the perpendicular dropped from the base line to the peak of I and J,

**Table for Calculation of A**
A is x-section area aorta for use in Starr's formula
$A = (SA \times a) - b$

| Age | a | b | Age | a | b |
|---|---|---|---|---|---|
| 20 | 1.20 | 0.1 | 47 | 2.25 | 0.45 |
| 21 | 1.25 | 0.1 | 48 | 2.30 | 0.50 |
| 22 | 1.30 | 0.1 | 49 | 2.35 | 0.55 |
| 23 | 1.35 | 0.1 | 50 | 2.40 | 0.60 |
| 24 | 1.40 | 0.1 | 51 | 2.45 | 0.65 |
| 25 | 1.40 | 0.1 | 52 | 2.50 | 0.70 |
| 26 | 1.40 | 0.2 | 53 | 2.55 | 0.75 |
| 27 | 1.45 | 0.2 | 54 | 2.60 | 0.80 |
| 28 | 1.50 | 0.2 | 55 | 2.65 | 0.80 |
| 29 | 1.55 | 0.2 | 56 | 2.70 | 0.80 |
| 30 | 1.60 | 0.2 | 57 | 2.75 | 0.85 |
| 31 | 1.60 | 0.2 | 58 | 2.80 | 0.90 |
| 32 | 1.60 | 0.2 | 59 | 2.90 | 0.95 |
| 33 | 1.65 | 0.2 | 60 | 3.00 | 1.0 |
| 34 | 1.70 | 0.2 | 61 | 3.05 | 1.05 |
| 35 | 1.75 | 0.25 | 62 | 3.1 | 1.1 |
| 36 | 1.80 | 0.30 | 63 | 3.15 | 1.2 |
| 37 | 1.85 | 0.30 | 64 | 3.20 | 1.3 |
| 38 | 1.90 | 0.30 | 65 | 3.25 | 1.35 |
| 39 | 1.95 | 0.30 | 66 | 3.30 | 1.40 |
| 40 | 2.00 | 0.30 | 67 | 3.35 | 1.50 |
| 41 | 2.05 | 0.30 | 68 | 3.40 | 1.60 |
| 42 | 2.10 | 0.30 | 69 | 3.50 | 1.70 |
| 43 | 2.10 | 0.35 | 70 | 3.60 | 1.80 |
| 44 | 2.10 | 0.40 | | | |
| 45 | 2.15 | 0.40 | | | |
| 46 | 2.20 | 0.40 | | | |

FIGURE 57. Table of a and b constants for calculation of A in Starr's formulae. (Starr, I., and Schroeder, H. A.: "Ballistocardiogram—Normal Standards, Abnormalities Commonly Found in Disease of Heart and Circulation, and Their Significance," *J. Clin. Investigation,* **19**:437, 1940.)

respectively (Figure 55, *B,* shaded areas). The base of the triangle is measured in seconds, and the altitude is measured in millimeters. The area can be computed from the formula: area = ½ bh, where b is the base in seconds, and h is the altitude in millimeters.

Cournand correlated the stroke volume as determined by the area formula and the catheter direct Fick method (*2*). He found a good correlation (18.5 per cent larger output by the Fick method), as is shown by Figure 60.

**Table of Values for Heart Rate and Cardiac Cycle for Use in Starr's Formula**

C = length of cardiac cycle, in seconds

| C | C 3/2 | Heart Rate | C | C 3/2 | Heart Rate |
|---|---|---|---|---|---|
| 1.501 | 1.84 | 40 | 0.723 | 0.615 | 83 |
| 1.464 | 1.772 | 41 | 0.714 | 0.603 | 84 |
| 1.428 | 1.709 | 42 | 0.706 | 0.593 | 85 |
| 1.396 | 1.65 | 43 | 0.697 | 0.583 | 86 |
| 1.364 | 1.594 | 44 | 0.689 | 0.572 | 87 |
| 1.334 | 1.541 | 45 | 0.682 | 0.564 | 88 |
| 1.305 | 1.491 | 46 | 0.674 | 0.554 | 89 |
| 1.277 | 1.444 | 47 | 0.667 | 0.545 | 90 |
| 1.252 | 1.400 | 48 | 0.659 | 0.535 | 91 |
| 1.225 | 1.365 | 49 | 0.652 | 0.527 | 92 |
| 1.201 | 1.316 | 50 | 0.645 | 0.518 | 93 |
| 1.177 | 1.277 | 51 | 0.638 | 0.510 | 94 |
| 1.155 | 1.241 | 52 | 0.631 | 0.502 | 95 |
| 1.132 | 1.206 | 53 | 0.625 | 0.494 | 96 |
| 1.112 | 1.172 | 54 | 0.618 | 0.486 | 97 |
| 1.092 | 1.142 | 55 | 0.612 | 0.479 | 98 |
| 1.072 | 1.111 | 56 | 0.606 | 0.472 | 99 |
| 1.053 | 1.082 | 57 | 0.600 | 0.465 | 100 |
| 1.035 | 1.054 | 58 | 0.594 | 0.458 | 101 |
| 1.017 | 1.026 | 59 | 0.588 | 0.451 | 102 |
| 1.000 | 1.000 | 60 | 0.582 | 0.444 | 103 |
| 0.9835 | 0.975 | 61 | 0.577 | 0.438 | 104 |
| 0.9675 | 0.952 | 62 | 0.571 | 0.432 | 105 |
| 0.9520 | 0.9295 | 63 | 0.566 | 0.426 | 106 |
| 0.9370 | 0.9080 | 64 | 0.561 | 0.420 | 107 |
| 0.9230 | 0.8861 | 65 | 0.555 | 0.410 | 108 |
| 0.9090 | 0.8660 | 66 | 0.551 | 0.408 | 109 |
| 0.895 | 0.848 | 67 | 0.545 | 0.403 | 110 |
| 0.882 | 0.828 | 68 | 0.540 | 0.398 | 111 |
| 0.869 | 0.810 | 69 | 0.536 | 0.392 | 112 |
| 0.857 | 0.794 | 70 | 0.531 | 0.387 | 113 |
| 0.845 | 0.777 | 71 | 0.526 | 0.382 | 114 |
| 0.833 | 0.755 | 72 | 0.522 | 0.377 | 115 |
| 0.822 | 0.745 | 73 | 0.517 | 0.372 | 116 |
| 0.811 | 0.731 | 74 | 0.513 | 0.367 | 117 |
| 0.800 | 0.716 | 75 | 0.508 | 0.362 | 118 |
| 0.789 | 0.701 | 76 | 0.504 | 0.358 | 119 |
| 0.779 | 0.687 | 77 | 0.500 | 0.353 | 120 |
| 0.769 | 0.674 | 78 | 0.496 | 0.349 | 121 |
| 0.766 | 0.661 | 79 | 0.491 | 0.344 | 122 |
| 0.750 | 0.649 | 80 | 0.488 | 0.341 | 123 |
| 0.741 | 0.638 | 81 | 0.484 | 0.336 | 124 |
| 0.731 | 0.626 | 82 | 0.480 | 0.332 | 125 |

FIGURE 58. Table of values for heart rate, cardiac cycle, and C 3/2 values used in Starr's formulae. (Starr, I., and Schroeder, H. A.: "Ballistocardiogram—Normal Standards, Abnormalities Commonly Found in Disease of Heart and Circulation, and Their Significance," *J. Clin. Investigation,* **19**:437, 1940.)

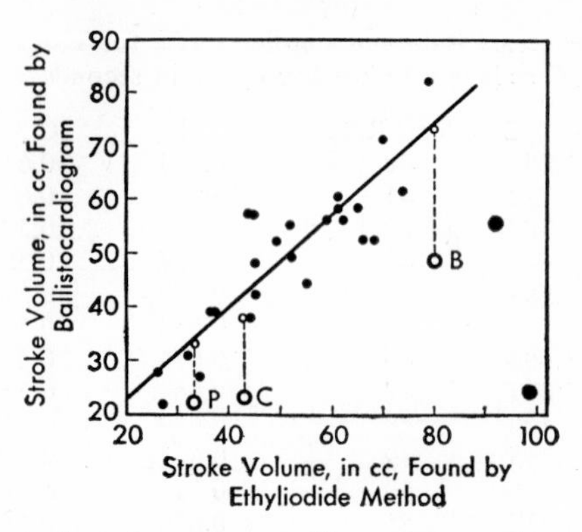


FIGURE 59. Comparison between cardiac stroke volume in cubic centimeters calculated from duplicate ballistocardiograms and from duplicate estimations by the improved ethyl iodide method. The small solid dots indicate that the ballistocardiographic records had the normal form. The line is the best line, regression y on x, for the 25 small solid dots. (Starr, I., Rawson, A. J., Schroeder, H. A., and Joseph, N. R.: "Studies on the Estimation of Cardiac Output in Man, and of Abnormalities in Cardiac Function, from the Heart's Recoil and the Blood's Impacts; the Ballistocardiogram," *Am. J. Physiol.*, **127**:1, 1939.)

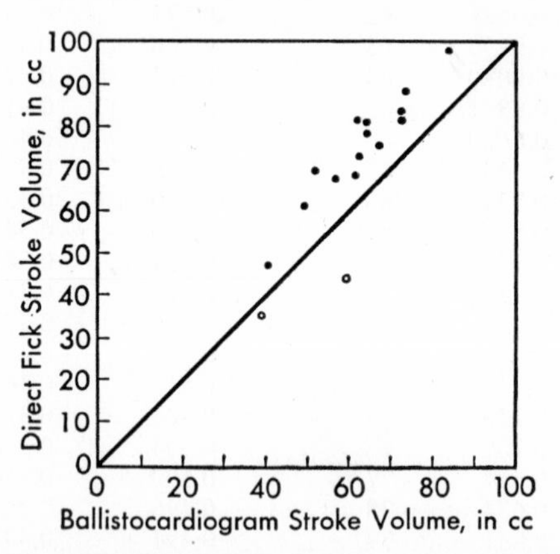


FIGURE 60. Sixteen individual measurements of stroke volume obtained by the direct Fick method plotted against the same measurements calculated from simultaneous ballistocardiographs. Open circles represent measurements in two subjects with rapid pulse, small and/or irregular ballistic complexes. Straight line is line of identity (see text). (Cournand, A., Ranges, H. A., and Riley, R. L.: "Comparison of Results of the Normal Ballistocardiogram and a Direct Fick Method in Measuring Cardiac Output in Man," *J. Clin. Investigation,* **21**:287, 1942.)

Other formulae derived by Starr for use in abnormal patterns were later discarded by him as unreliable (*1*).

It became evident that the use of the cross-sectional area of the aorta was unnecessary, and that it implied that the forces that occurred in the pulmonary circuit were not significant in the production of the IJ stroke. This last is not the case (see above). Therefore, Tanner (*4*), working with Starr's original data, devised a new formula which does not use the area of the aorta: $SV = 100\sqrt{(2 \text{ area I} + \text{Area J})\ C\ 1/2}$, where 100 is the constant necessary to bring the results up to Cournand's mean catheter figures. Tanner felt that these results are probably too high, and that a constant of 60 would probably give figures which are nearer the truth, since a patient with a catheter in the heart is not likely to be in a basal condition.

Tanner also described the reliability of the ballistocardiographic method in general. He states that the coefficient of reliability of the ballistocardiogram is 0.91. He further states that, according to Nickerson (*3*) and Warren (*8*), the catheter method is slightly less reliable. Correcting for the reliability of the two methods involved, Tanner states that the coefficient of correlation for Starr's data (amplitude formula versus ethyl iodide technique) is 0.96. Treating Cournand's figures in the same manner (area formula versus catheter-Fick method) results in a correlation greater than 0.95.

Using Tanner's area formula, Paine and Schock recently reported upon the variability of the cardiac output determinations made from the ballistocardiogram (*9*). Their results show good relationship between different observations on the same trace made by the same observer (Figure 61, *A*) and different observations made on the same trace by different observers (Figure 61, *B*). They further demonstrated that the cardiac output rises with a meal (Figure 62, *A*), but that it does not change significantly after 1 min rest on the table (Figure 62, *B*).

In 1946, Molomut reported the use of a simplified formula (after Starr) with a high-frequency table to determine relative changes in cardiac output (*10*).

The formula utilized the height of the I and J valleys in millimeters and the cycle length in seconds, as follows: $SV = \sqrt{(I + J)\ C\ 3/2}$.

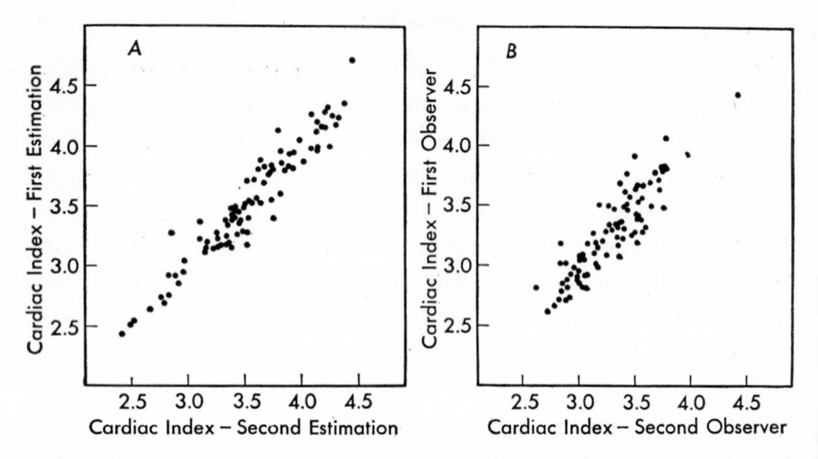


FIGURE 61. (*A*) Scatter plot of duplicate determinations by the same observer from different respiratory cycles of the same record. Mean of first estimations = 3.56. Mean of second estimations = 3.54. N = 90. Correlation coefficient = 0.93. Standard error of estimate = 0.168 L/min/M 2. (B) Scatter plot of duplicate determinations by different observers from different respiratory cycles of the same record. Mean of first observer = 3.65. Mean of second observer = 3.68. N = 90. Correlation coefficient = 0.91. Standard error of estimate = 0.191 L/min/M 2. (Paine, R. M., and Schock, N. W.: "The Variability of Cardiac Output Estimation Made with the High Frequency Undamped Ballistocardiogram," *Circulation,* **1**:1026, 1950.)

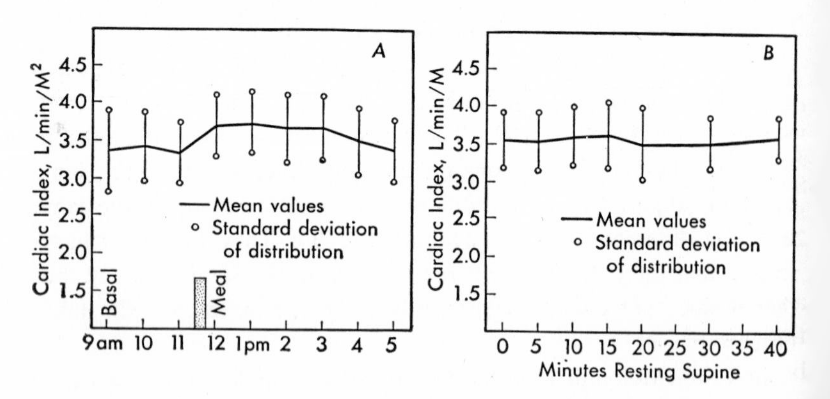


FIGURE 62. (*A*) Mean cardiac index of 20 subjects who were basal at 9:00 A.M., ambulatory thereafter, and who ingested a standard meal at 11:30 A.M. The elevation from 12:00 to 3:00 P.M. is significant. (*B*) Mean cardiac index of 10 subjects resting supine. Determinations made within 1 min after reclining did not differ significantly from those made

This formula gives arbitrary figures which are useful in determining relative cardiac output or changes in output.

The formulae described above are for use with a table similar to Starr's high-frequency table.

Nickerson devised a formula for use with his low-frequency damped table which is a modification of that first discussed by him in 1945 (*3*). It is:

$$SV = \frac{5.02 \ F \times P}{T \times L} \ ml$$

In this formula F is determined, as illustrated in Figure 63, by measuring the distance between the peak of the first major footward deflection (I) and the peak of the first major headward deflection (J)

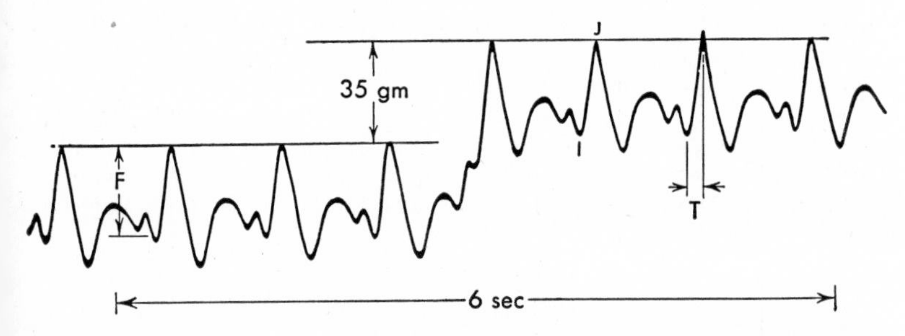


FIGURE 63. Ballistocardiogram taken with Nickerson's low-frequency damped table. The figure demonstrates the method of calibration and indicates the measurements to be taken from the tracing. (Nickerson, J. L., Warren, J. W., and Brannon, E. S.: "The Cardiac Output in Man; Studies with the Low Frequency, Critically-damped Ballistocardiograph, and the Method of Right Atrial Catheterization," *J. Clin. Investigation,* **26**:1, 1947.)

and making a simple proportionality calculation related to the deviation effected by the known weight of 35 gm applied to the foot of the ballistic bed during the tracing. T is the time interval between the peak of the first footward movement (I) and the peak of the first major headward movement (J). The quantity L is the height of the

in the following 40 min. (Paine, R. M., and Schock, N. W.: "The Variability of Cardiac Output Estimation Made with the High Frequency Undamped Ballistocardiogram," *Circulation,* **1**:1026, 1950.)

subject in centimeters, and the factor 5.02 is a constant which adjusts the ballistic results to best fit the catheter data used in the determination of the Fick technique. The factor **P** may be obtained from Figure 64, and it equals the square root of the arithmetic mean of

| Pa | $\sqrt{Pa}$ | P | Pa | $\sqrt{Pa}$ | P |
|---|---|---|---|---|---|
| 50 | 7.1 | 5.0 | 100 | 10.0 | 10.0 |
| 52 | 7.2 | 5.3 | 102 | 10.1 | 10.1 |
| 54 | 7.3 | 5.6 | 104 | 10.2 | 10.2 |
| 56 | 7.5 | 5.8 | 106 | 10.3 | 10.3 |
| 58 | 7.6 | 6.1 | 108 | 10.4 | 10.4 |
| 60 | 7.7 | 6.4 | 110 | 10.5 | 10.5 |
| 62 | 7.9 | 6.7 | 112 | 10.6 | 10.6 |
| 64 | 8.0 | 7.0 | 114 | 10.7 | 10.7 |
| 66 | 8.1 | 7.2 | 116 | 10.8 | 10.8 |
| 68 | 8.2 | 7.5 | 118 | 10.9 | 10.9 |
| 70 | 8.4 | 7.8 | 120 | 11.0 | 11.0 |
| 72 | 8.5 | 8.1 | 122 | 11.0 | 11.0 |
| 74 | 8.6 | 8.3 | 124 | 11.1 | 11.1 |
| 76 | 8.7 | 8.5 | 126 | 11.2 | 11.2 |
| 78 | 8.8 | 8.7 | 128 | 11.3 | 11.3 |
| 80 | 8.9 | 8.9 | 130 | 11.4 | 11.4 |
| 82 | 9.1 | 9.1 | 132 | 11.5 | 11.5 |
| 84 | 9.2 | 9.2 | 134 | 11.6 | 11.6 |
| 86 | 9.3 | 9.3 | 136 | 11.7 | 11.7 |
| 88 | 9.4 | 9.4 | 138 | 11.7 | 11.7 |
| 90 | 9.5 | 9.5 | 140 | 11.8 | 11.8 |
| 92 | 9.6 | 9.6 | 142 | 11.9 | 11.9 |
| 94 | 9.7 | 9.7 | 144 | 12.0 | 12.0 |
| 96 | 9.8 | 9.8 | | | |
| 98 | 9.9 | 9.9 | | | |

FIGURE 64. Values for the factor P in Nickerson's formula. (Nickerson, J. L., Warren, J. W., and Brannon, E. S.: "The Cardiac Output in Man; Studies with the Low Frequency, Critically-damped Ballistocardiograph, and the Method of Right Atrial Catheterization," *J. Clin. Investigation,* **26**:1, 1947.)

the systolic and the diastolic pressures over the range of most of the blood pressures encountered. At mean pressures below 80, the results using the square root of Pa (arithmetic mean) were too large, and lower P values were empirically derived. Using this technique Nicker-

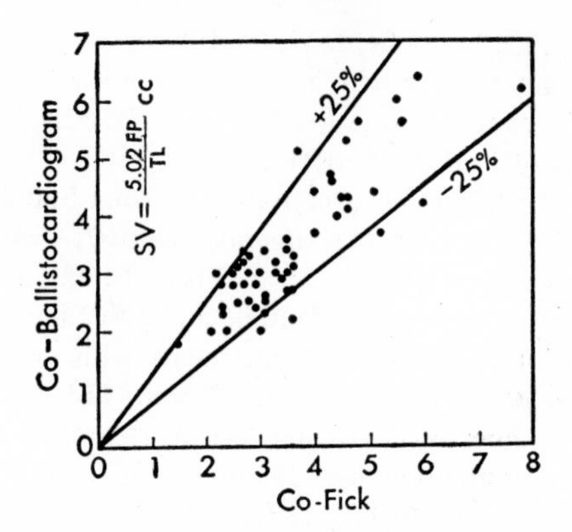


FIGURE 65. A comparison of the cardiac output values using Nickerson's technique as compared with the direct Fick procedure. The limits of ± 25 per cent deviation from the catheter values are shown. (Nickerson, J. L., Warren, J. W., and Brannon, E. S.: "The Cardiac Output in Man; Studies with the Low Frequency, Critically-damped Ballistocardiograph, and the Method of Right Atrial Catheterization," *J. Clin. Investigation,* **26**:1, 1947.)

son was able to show that 87 per cent of the values obtained by the ballistic method of calculation fall within 25 per cent of those by the catheter method (Figure 65). The correlation coefficient relating the data from the two methods is 0.83. According to Tanner (*4*), this figure becomes 0.95 when the two methods used are corrected for "unreliability."

## REFERENCES

### CARDIAC OUTPUT

1. STARR, I., RAWSON, A. J., SCHROEDER, H. A., and JOSEPH, N. R.: "Studies on the Estimation of Cardiac Output in Man, and of Abnormalities in Cardiac Function, from the Heart's Recoil and the Blood's Impacts; the Ballistocardiogram," *Am. J. Physiol.,* **127**:1, 1939.
2. COURNAND, A., RANGES, H. A., and RILEY, R. L.: "Comparison of Results of the Normal Ballistocardiogram and a Direct Fick Method in Measuring Cardiac Output in Man," *J. Clin. Investigation,* **21**:287, 1942.

3. NICKERSON, J. L., WARREN, J. W., and BRANNON, E. S.: "The Cardiac Output in Man; Studies with the Low Frequency, Critically-damped Ballistocardiograph, and the Method of Right Atrial Catheterization," *J. Clin. Investigation,* **26**:1, 1947.
4. TANNER, J. M.: "The Construction of Normal Standards for Cardiac Output in Man," *J. Clin. Investigation,* **28**:567, 1949.
5. BAZETT, H. C., COTTON, F. S., LAPLAS, L. B., and SCOTT, J. B.: "The Calculation of Cardiac Output and Effective Peripheral Resistance from Blood Pressure Measurements with an Appendix on the Size of the Aorta in Man," *Am. J. Physiol.,* **113**:312, 1935.
6. SUTER, F.: "Ueber das Verhalten des Aortenumfanges unter physiologischen und pathologischen Bedingungen," *Arch. f. Exper. Path. Anat. u. Pharmakol.,* **39**:289, 1897.
7. DREYER, G., RAY, W., and WALKER, E. W. A.: "The Size of the Aorta in Warm-Blooded Animals and Its Relationship to the Body Weight and to the Surface Area Expressed in a Formula," *Proc. Roy. Soc. (London),* Series *B,* **86**:39, 1912.
8. WARREN, J. W., STEAD, E. A., JR., and BRANNON, E. S.: "The Cardiac Output in Man; A Study of Some of the Errors in the Method of Right Heart Catheterization," *Am. J. Physiol.,* **145**:458, 1946.
9. PAINE, R. M., and SCHOCK, N. W.: "The Variability of Cardiac Output Estimation Made with the High Frequency Undamped Ballistocardiogram," *Circulation,* **1**:1026, 1950.
10. MOLOMUT, N., and ALLEN, S. C.: "Effect of Pressure Breathing on Circulation at High Altitude as Measured by the Ballistocardiograph," *J. Aviation Med.,* **16–17**:350, 1945–1946.

CHAPTER SIX

# Respiratory Variation of the Ballistocardiogram

THE empirical observation of the respiratory variation of the ballistocardiogram was probably first reported by Heald and Tucker in 1922 (*1*). It has since been described by other authors (*2, 3,* and *4*).

Respiration affects the ballistocardiogram in at least two ways: it changes the position of the heart with respect to the long axis of the body—as the diaphragm rises with expiration, the heart becomes more lateral; and it produces changes in blood flow to and from the right and left heart—inspiration increases venous return to the right heart by diminishing intrapleural pressure at the same time that it decreases venous return to the left heart; the reverse occurs with expiration. A detailed account of the effects of respiration on the component parts of the ballistocardiogram follows.

If the apex thrust causes the H-wave, then the more lateral the heart, the more effective the vertical component of the apex thrust will be in producing the H-wave. Since the heart becomes more lateral in expiration, one would expect the H-wave to increase in expiration. This expiratory increase occurred in 55 per cent of 40 adult normals (20 males and 20 females) (Figure 66). However, inspiration increases the total volume of the heart (*5*) and therefore it is likely that the total force of the apex thrust is increased with inspiration. Furthermore, the auricular component of the H-wave probably increases with inspiration, since the venous return to the right heart increases with inspiration. This would tend to counteract the effect of the change in position and may account for the number of subjects where the H-wave either showed no change or increased with inspiration.

| | H-Wave | Per Cent | | I-Wave | Per Cent |
|---|---|---|---|---|---|
| Decreased | 14 Males<br>8 Females | 55 | Decreased | 0 Males<br>1 Female | 2.5 |
| Increased | 5 Males<br>10 Females | 37.5 | Increased | 20 Males<br>14 Females | 85 |
| No Change | 2 Males<br>1 Female | 7.5 | No Change | 1 Male<br>4 Females | 12.5 |
| | J-Wave | | | K-Wave | |
| Decreased | 0 Males<br>0 Females | 0 | Decreased | 2 Males<br>1 Female | 7.5 |
| Increased | 19 Males<br>20 Females | 97.5 | Increased | 16 Males<br>16 Females | 82.5 |
| No Change | 1 Male | 2.5 | No Change | 2 Males<br>2 Females | 10 |

FIGURE 66. Variation of H- I- J- K waves with inspiration—20 males, 20 females.

If the I-wave is produced by cardiac recoil, then one would expect to find normal individuals whose I valley is deeper in inspiration than in expiration, since the footward component of the cardiac recoil is more pronounced when the heart is more vertical, i.e., in inspiration. Figure 45, *A,* arrow 1 as compared with arrow 2, shows examples of this inspiratory increase of the I-wave which occurred in 85 per cent of 40 normal adults (Figure 66). Another cause for the increased HI stroke in inspiration might be deduced from the experiments reported by Boyd and Patras (5) which show that the combined diastolic filling and combined stroke volumes of left and right heart are greater in inspiration. One would therefore expect that the effect of heart recoil would be greater in inspiration.

Inspection of 40 normal ballistocardiograms revealed that in 39 out of 40 cases the J peak was greater in inspiration than in expiration (Figure 66). (Figure 45, *B, C,* and *D,* note arrows.) The increased IJ stroke in inspiration is probably related to the changes in stroke volumes with respiration and may be explained in the following manner:

In 1942, Shuler and co-workers confirmed the findings of Boyd and Patras and further showed that, although the total ventricular volume increased with inspiration, the left ventricular stroke volume decreased (*6*). They also showed that the right heart stroke volume variations were greater than those of the left heart. Because of this, the total stroke volume variation parallels that of the right heart (Figure 67). This was further illustrated by Starr (7) who reversed

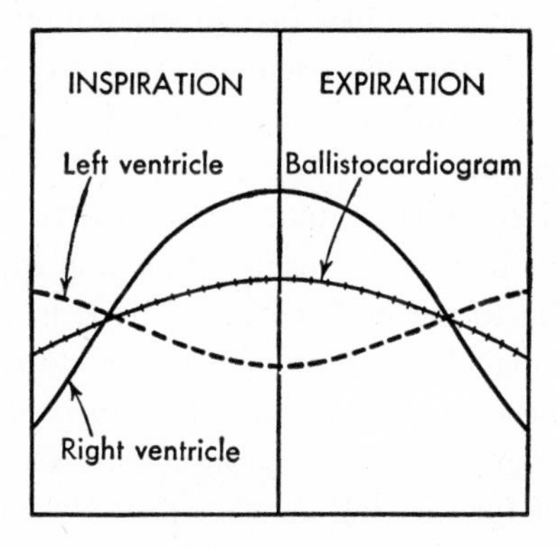


FIGURE 67. Drawing comparing the respiratory variation of the ventricular stroke volumes [after Shuler *et al.*, (6)] with the ballistocardiogram stroke volume variation. Note that the right heart variation is greater than the left; the variation of the total stroke volume will therefore increase with inspiration, thus paralleling the ballistocardiogram stroke volume (see text). (Brown, H. R., Jr., and deLalla, V., Jr.: "The Ballistocardiogram, Description and Clinical Use," *Am. J. Med.*, **9**:718, 1950.)

the IJ stroke respiratory variation when he reversed the right heart respiratory variation by forcing inspiration with intermittent positive-pressure breathing. These findings confirm the theory that the IJ stroke is proportional to the total stroke volume and is caused by forces occurring in the pulmonary circuit as well as the greater systemic circulation.

The fact that left heart stroke volume increased in expiration, while the right heart output decreases, may be understood and deduced when one considers the effect of expiration upon the venous return to the left and right auricles. Expiration increases the intrapleural (intrathoracic) pressure. The increased intrapleural pressure impedes the return of systemic venous blood to the right auricle, while it increases the return of pulmonary blood to the left auricle. The ventricles can only eject as much blood as they get, and one would therefore expect the right heart stroke volume to decrease simultaneously with a left heart increase (during expiration).

The respiratory variation is exaggerated (increased) in certain pathological states. When the IJ amplitude in expiration is approximately one half (or less) than that in inspiration, it can be stated almost unequivocally that the respiratory variation is abnormal. For doubtful cases a quantitative means of measuring the respiratory variation can be used.

The total relative cardiac output measurements of both stroke and minute volume can be made in inspiration and in expiration by applying Starr's formula to the proper beats (*8*). It is apparent from the above discussion that the inspiratory total minute volume figures will be higher than the expiratory figures. This variation may be termed the "ballistocardiogram respiratory variation." One of us (V.deL.) devised a method for arriving at what may be called the "ballistocardiogram respiratory variation index," which falls into certain limiting figures for the normal adult (*4*).

The ballistocardiogram respiratory variation index is determined in the following manner: pick the smallest expiratory and the largest inspiratory beats in several consecutive respirations. This tends to reduce errors of choice. The measurements made on the expiratory beats are used to calculate the expiratory stroke and minute volumes, while the measurements made on the inspiratory beats are used to calculate the inspiratory stroke and minute volumes.

Measure in millimeters the depth of the I valley below the base line and the height of the J peak above the base line (or use the respective areas under each wave in the "area" formula) for expiratory and inspiratory beats. C for use in either height or area formula of Starr is computed on the basis of the cycle length between the beat preceding the one measured and the one actually measured. Thus, if beat 2 is to be used, C will be the cycle length between beats 1 and 2

This was decided upon in order to obtain a better approximation of the actual inspiratory and expiratory stroke volumes, since the cycle length (and therefore the filling time) varies with respiration (*9*). These different heart rates are used to calculate the inspiratory and expiratory minute volumes, respectively. The inspiratory minute volume figure assumes that the heart continues to beat at the inspiratory rate for 1 min, and the same with expiration.

Subtracting the expiratory figure from the inspiratory figure gives the total respiratory variation in cubic centimeters per minute. Dividing this by the surface area in square meters gives the respiratory variation index (Figure 68).

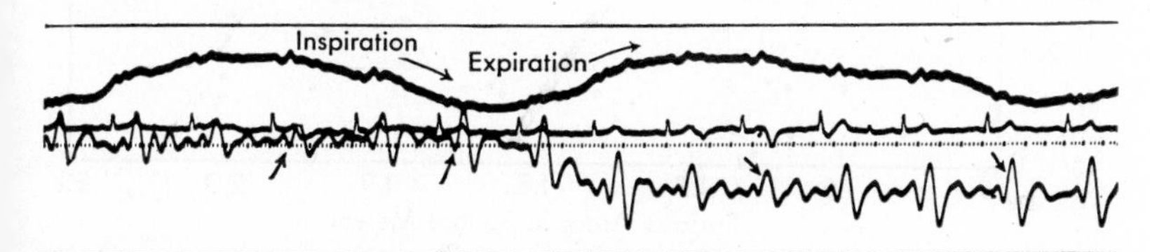


FIGURE 68. A record of an adult man. The expiratory minute volume was computed from measurements made on expiratory beats (first and third arrows); the inspiratory minute volume was computed from measurement made on inspiratory beats (second and fourth arrows). In computing the index for actual use at least four and usually six consecutive respirations are used, with equal numbers on each side of the standardization. (Brown, H. R., Jr., and deLalla, V., Jr.: "The Ballistocardiogram, Description and Clinical Use," *Am. J. Med.*, **9**:718, 1950.)

A (when used) and K are derived in the manner described under the section on cardiac output. They will have the same value for both the expiratory and inspiratory calculations. Since this is so, it should be possible to set up other normal standards using a simple method of measuring the respiratory variation of the IJ stroke which would not necessarily represent the actual variation in cubic centimeters per minute; for instance, the ratio of inspiratory IJ to expiratory IJ probably has normal limiting factors; it remains but to determine what the normal limits are. In many clinical applications this ratio would be just as useful as the actual determination outlined above.

The respiratory variation index of 50 normal adults between the

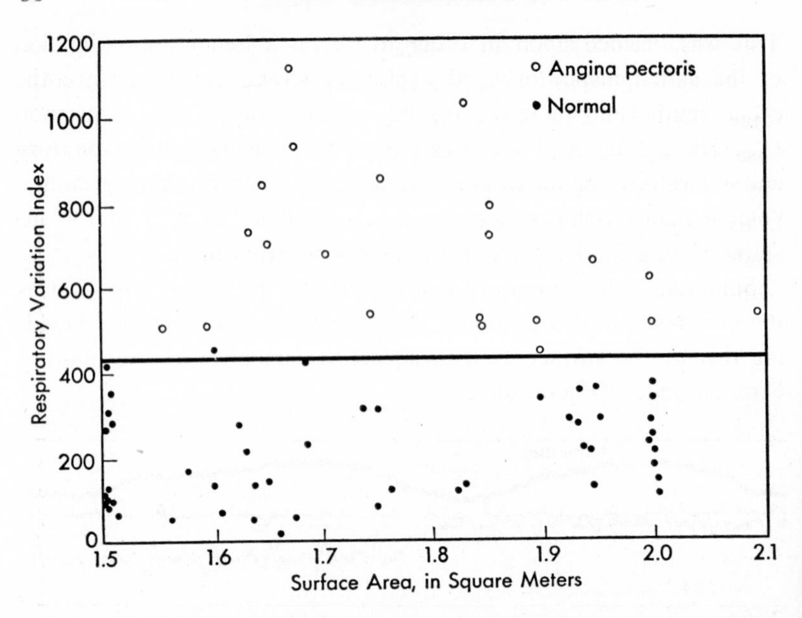


FIGURE 69. A graph of the respiratory variation index against surface area. The solid points beneath the line (at 450 on the index scale) represent normal men and women from 20 to 69 years of age. The open circles above the 480 index line represent patients with angina pectoris (see text). (Brown, H. R., Jr., and deLalla, V., Jr.: "The Ballistocardiogram, Description and Clinical Use," *Am. J. Med.*, **9**:718, 1950.)

ages of 20 and 70 has been measured using Starr's original formula (*4*). The results are shown by Figure 69. Note that although the index tends to increase with surface area, with one exception, all normals are below 450, and all but 3 fall below 400. It must be stated that the bulk of the series were between the ages of 25 and 35. However, some normals within the older age groups are included, and thus far, all those measured are within the limits described above.

The variation of the K-wave with respiration appears to be a paradox; since the left ventricular output and systemic blood pressure drop with inspiration, one would expect the JK stroke to be less in inspiration (since it is produced by deceleration of the impulse wave in the legs). However, measurement of the JK stroke showed that it increased in length in inspiration in 32 out of 40 normals (Figure 66)

This is an apparent increase rather than a real increase, since the JK stroke is affected by the height of the J peak as well as by other forces. The higher the J peak, the greater the return swing toward the base line will be, and the longer the JK stroke. A true estimate of the K valley can be obtained by determining the ratio of the IJ stroke to the JK stroke. When this ratio is measured, the effect of the J peak tends to be eliminated, and it is found that the IJ/JK ratio decreases with expiration (i.e., there is a greater "true" K-wave in expiration).

## REFERENCES

### RESPIRATORY VARIATION

1. Heald, C. B., and Tucker, W. S.: "The Recoil Curves as Shown by the Hot Wire Microphone," *Proc. Roy. Soc. (London),* Series *B,* **93**:281, 1922.
2. Starr, I., and Friedlan, C.: "On Cause of Respiratory Variation of Ballistocardiogram with Note on Sinus Arrhythmia," *J. Clin. Investigation,* **25**:53, 1946.
3. deLalla, V., Jr., and Brown, H. R., Jr.: "The Respiratory Variation of the Ballistocardiogram," *Am. J. Med.,* **9**:728, 1950.
4. Brown, H. R., Jr., and deLalla, V., Jr.: "The Ballistocardiogram, Description and Clinical Use," *Am. J. Med.,* **9**:718, 1950.
5. Boyd, T. C., and Patras, M.: "Variations in Filling and Output of Ventricles with Phases of Respiration," *Am. J. Physiol.,* **134**:74, 1941.
6. Shuler, R., Ensor, C., Gunning, R., Moss, W., and Johnson, V.: "Differential Effects of Respiration on Left and Right Ventricles," *Am. J. Physiol.,* **137**:602, 1942.
7. Starr, I., and Schroeder, H. A.: "Ballistocardiogram—Normal Standards, Abnormalities Commonly Found in Disease of Heart and Circulation, and Their Significance," *J. Clin. Investigation,* **19**:437, 1940.
8. Starr, I., Rawson, A. J., Schroeder, H. A., and Joseph, N. R.: "Studies on the Estimation of Cardiac Output in Man, and of Abnormalities in Cardiac Function, from the Heart's Recoil and the Blood's Impacts; the Ballistocardiogram," *Am. J. Physiol.,* **127**:1, 1939.
9. deLalla, V., Jr., and Brown, H. R., Jr.: "Normal Respiratory Variation of Cycle Length, QT Interval, and Corrected QT Interval of the Electrocardiogram," *Am. Heart J.,* **39**:519, 1950.

PART TWO

# ABNORMAL SECTION

CHAPTER SEVEN

# Significance of Normal and Abnormal Patterns

IT IS the purpose of this section to show in what ways abnormal ballistocardiograms differ from normal, and to demonstrate how these differences may be used in the diagnosis and evaluation of various clinical states. However, it is essential that one does not create ballistocardiographic heart disease where there is none. The full limits of a "normal pattern" have yet to be defined, and the significance of certain deviations from the "normal," such as an increased respiratory variation, are not fully understood. Investigations along these lines are most important, and a fuller clinical application of the ballistocardiogram awaits their completion.

Before detailed analysis of a ballistocardiogram can be undertaken, a standard method of procuring the traces must be worked out. It is evident that the subject must approach basal conditions, and that the technique must allow for a reasonable "rest period" on the table. One such system follows:

1. Records should be taken before meals, preferably before breakfast.
2. Ascertain that no tight abdominal supports are being worn.
3. Take initial record at once, together with immediate blood-pressure readings.
4. After 15 min rest, take second ballistocardiogram and second blood-pressure reading.
5. Record patient's weight, height, and age, as well as clinical data.

An important part of the clinical use of the ballistocardiogram is the proper appraisal of the normal pattern; by this, we do not mean merely the recognition of a normal pattern, but rather, what does a normal pattern mean in terms of cardiovascular heart disease?

It must be recognized that a normal pattern does not rule out heart disease. However, the generalization can be made that a normal pattern implies good cardiac muscle function under the conditions at the time of the record. This implication is a statement of probability, and several other "probability statements" can be made:

1. A normal ballistocardiogram is excellent evidence against low-output congestive failure but does not rule out those conditions which produce high-output failure such as hyperthyroidism, anemia, arteriovenous aneurysm, etc.

2. A normal ballistocardiogram is good evidence against a recent myocardial infarction.

3. A normal ballistocardiogram is excellent evidence against hypertensive heart disease; it does not exclude hypertensive vascular disease.

4. A normal ballistocardiogram is good evidence against angina pectoris.

5. A normal pattern does not rule out valvular lesions of any character or etiology but is evidence against aortic stenosis.

6. A normal pattern is evidence against conditions which, if present, would impair cardiac muscular efficiency, i.e., constrictive pericarditis, severe myocarditis, beriberi heart disease, etc.

7. A normal pattern does not rule out congenital heart disease.

The descriptions of the normal can be applied to the abnormal. Each tracing can be studied from the point of view of amplitude, regularity, definitiveness, variations of H-I-J-K waves, the respiratory variation, and H-K times (Figure 70).

Low amplitude of pattern may occur in any situation where the output is low and/or the ventricular muscle is weak (Figures 71 and 72).

In general, irregularity and indefinitiveness of pattern indicate serious impairment of ventricular function, such as might occur with infarction, congestive heart failure, pericarditis, or myocarditis (Figure 72).

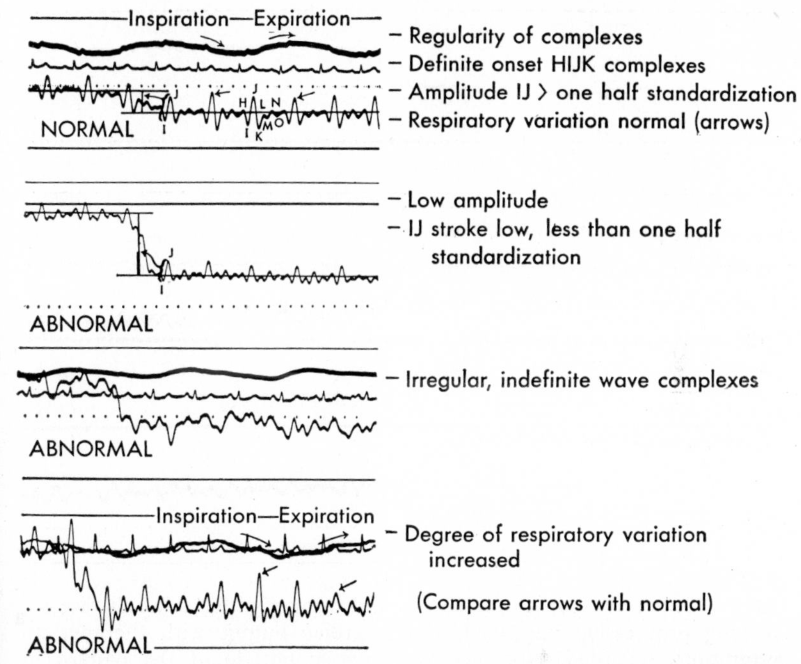


FIGURE 70. A comparison of a normal ballistocardiogram (top record) with three abnormal records. The normal record is characterized by regularity and definitiveness of pattern. Note that the height of the IJ stroke is more than one half the change in base line caused by the standardization (see text). There is a respiratory variation of the height of the IJ stroke, but it is not marked (arrows).

The first abnormal record demonstrates an abnormally low amplitude of the IJ stroke; the height of the IJ stroke is less than half the standardization.

The second abnormal record demonstrates what is meant by "irregular, indefinite wave patterns." Note that the pattern characteristics change from beat to beat (irregularity), and that the onset of each wave pattern cannot be readily determined (indefinitiveness).

The third abnormal record shows a marked respiratory variation of the height of the IJ stroke produced by an abnormal expiratory wave pattern. Compare the expiratory and inspiratory beats with the normal (arrows). (Brown, H. R., Jr., and deLalla, V., Jr.: "The Ballistocardiogram, Description and Clinical Use," *Am. J. Med.,* **9**:718, 1950.)

More specific changes with abnormalities of individual waves occur in such conditions as hypotension (Figure 73, *A*), hypertension

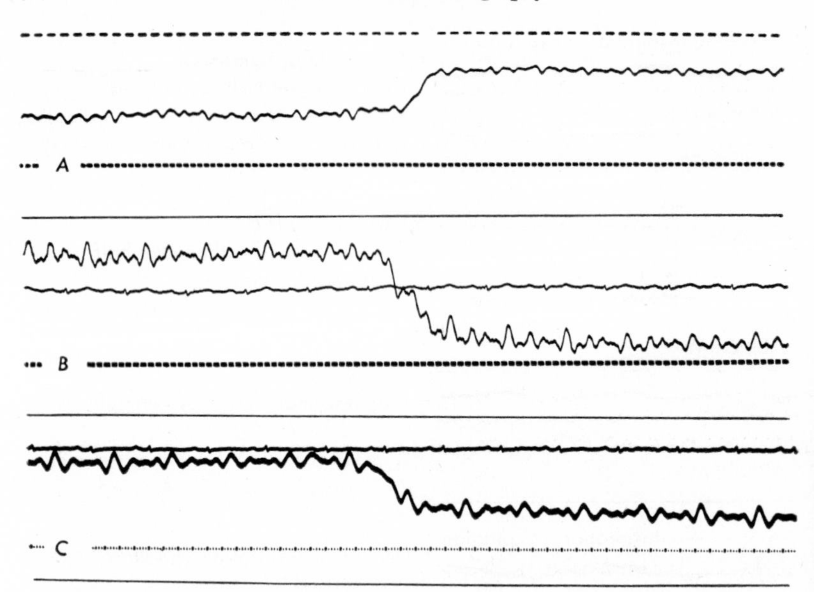


FIGURE 71. Serial records of a 39-year-old woman with Addison's disease, showing progressive improvement of cardiac output with therapy, no respirations recorded. Note the very low amplitude of the pattern in tracing *A* at a time when patient was experiencing crises. Record *B* was taken 6 weeks later, after daily doses of 10 to 15 cc of adrenal cortical extract. Record *C* was taken 6 months later. Note the improved output as reflected by the increased amplitude.

(Figure 73, *B*), coarctation of the aorta (Figure 73, *C*), healed myocardial infarction (Figure 74), and aortic stenosis (Figure 74).

Abnormal (i.e., increased) respiratory variation occurs particularly with coronary artery disease (Figure 75) but also may be seen with other conditions, such as hypertension (Figure 77, *A*), postsympathectomy (Figure 77, *B*), pulmonary emphysema (Figure 78), and in normal subjects during resistance breathing (Figure 75) or when subjected to cold (Figure 75).

The respiratory variation index has been measured in cases of clinically diagnosed coronary insufficiency with normal blood pressure and without coronary occlusion. It was found that the index was higher than 450 in all cases (see Chapter 8).

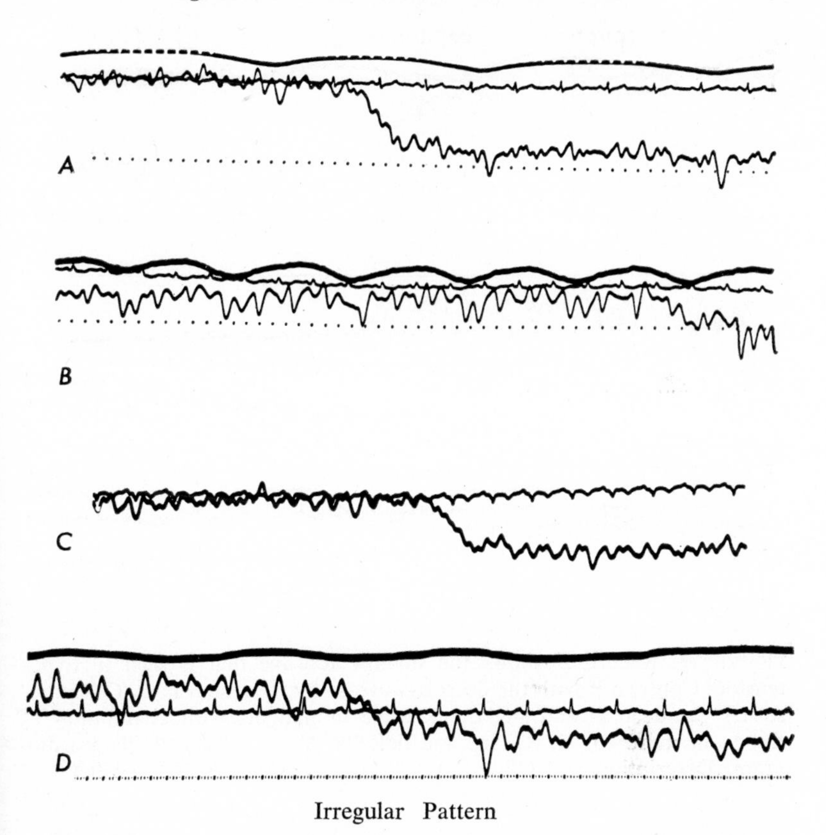


Irregular Pattern

FIGURE 72. Four patterns demonstrating irregularity, indefinitiveness, and low amplitude of pattern: (*A*) taken on a patient 2 weeks following an acute myocardial infarction, (*B*) a record of a patient with acute tuberculous pericarditis, (*C*) tracing of a patient with acute severe rheumatic myocarditis, (*D*) a record of a patient in congestive cardiac failure.

Variation of the H-K time usually is present in those instances where the pattern is irregular and indefinite, i.e., infarction, failure, or myocarditis (Figure 72).

Figure 76 summarizes the findings in various conditions.

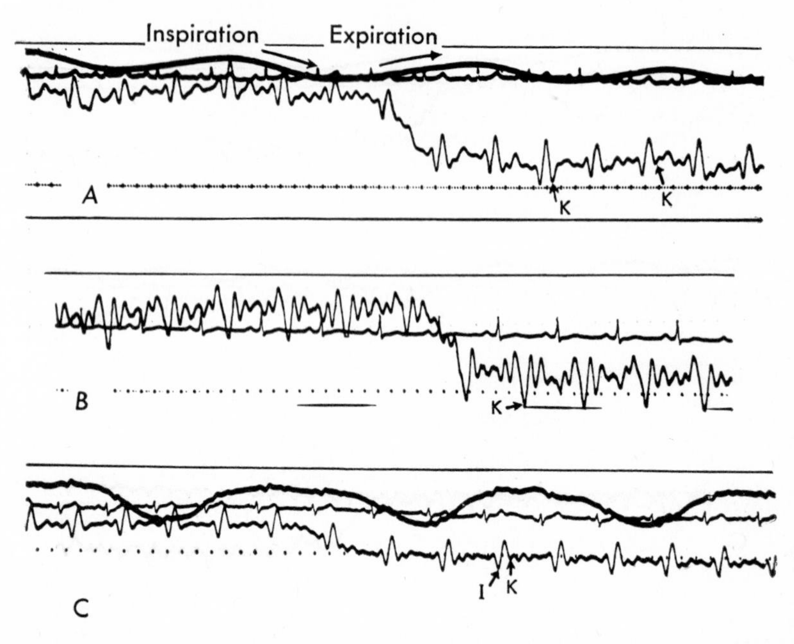


FIGURE 73. Record *A* shows the shallow K-wave that is seen in hypotension. Contrast it with the deep K-wave of hypertension in *B*. *C* demonstrates the deep I- and shallow K-wave in patients with coarctation of the aorta. (Brown, H. R., Jr., and deLalla, V., Jr.: "The Ballistocardiogram, Description and Clinical Use," *Am. J. Med.,* **9**:718, 1950.)

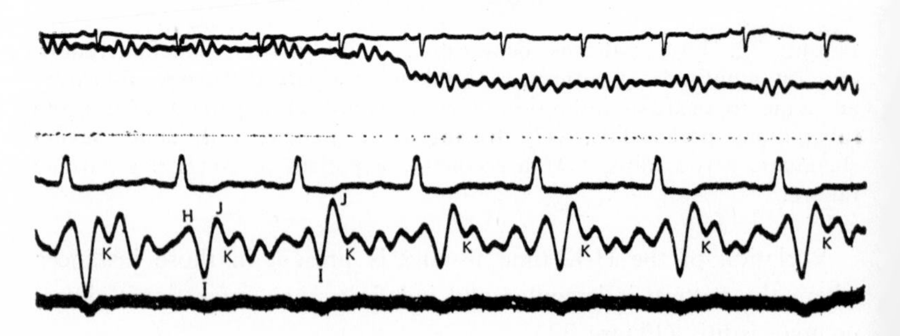


FIGURE 74. The upper record shows the M-type pattern caused by high H, low I, and high L peaks, frequently seen following coronary occlusions. The lower record shows the deep I- and shallow K-wave in the tracing of a patient with aortic stenosis.

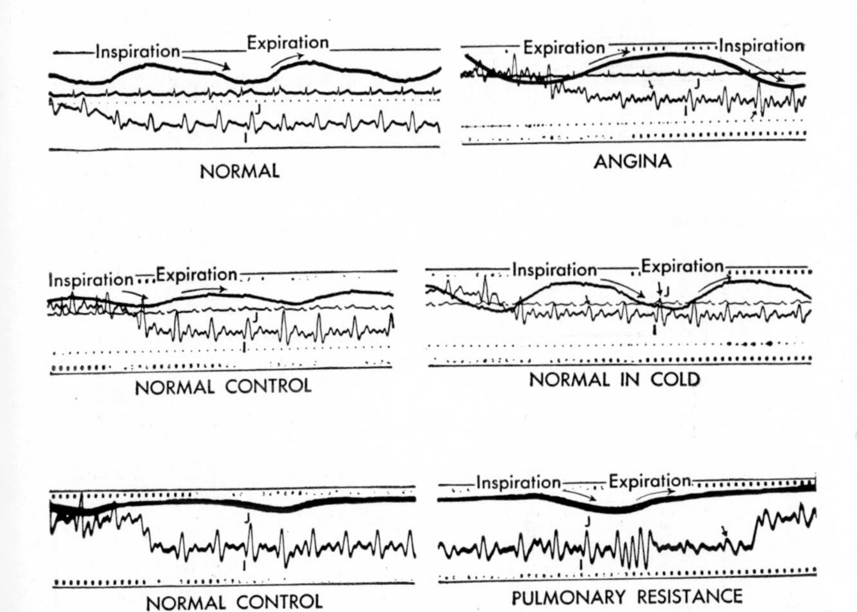


FIGURE 75. Six tracings comparing normals (left-hand records) with coronary insufficiency (upper right record), normal suddenly exposed to cold of 60°F (middle right record), and normal breathing through a resistance (lowest right record). The middle records are on the same normal male adult, before exposure to cold (left-hand record) and after 1 min of exposure to cold (right-hand record). The two lowest records are similarly on the same normal male adult before (right-hand record) and 30 sec after resistance breathing was started (left-hand record). Note the similarity of pattern in each of the right-hand records: increased respiratory variation, with the shallow I- and deep K-waves appearing in expiration (arrows). (deLalla, V., Jr., and Brown, H. R., Jr.: "The Respiratory Variation of the Ballistocardiogram," *Am. J. Med.,* **9**:728, 1950.)

## Summary Chart—Ballistocardiogram Changes in Disease

| *Diagnosis* | *Amplitude* | *Pattern Regularity* | *Complexes Well Defined* | *Respiratory Variation* | *H-I-J-K Strokes* | *H-K Time* | *Remarks* |
|---|---|---|---|---|---|---|---|
| Hypertensive vascular disease | Usually normal; may be low | Regular | Well defined | May be increased | Deep K | Constant | Suspect coarctation of aorta when BP high with normal or shallow K-waves |
| Hypertensive cardiovascular disease | Low | Variable | Variable | Usually increased | K usually deep; I shallow; high IJ take-off | Constant | With failure, pattern may become irregular and indefinite |
| Myocardial infarction a. 24 to 48 hr | Variable | May be irregular | May be indefinite | Increased | Usually abnormal | Variable | Will partly depend on previous infarction, etc. |
| b. 2 to 6 weeks | Variable | May be irregular | May be indefinite | Usually increased | May see M-shaped complexes with high N-waves, especially in expiration | Variable | Varies with progress of healing |
| c. 1 to 9 years | Variable | Variable | Variable | May be increased | Often many M-shaped complexes | Constant or inconstant | Pattern may be entirely normal |
| Coronary insufficiency | Usually slightly low | Regular | Definite | Increased RVI 450 | May be normal; sometimes high H in expiration | | |

|  |  |  |  |  |  |  |  |
|---|---|---|---|---|---|---|---|
| Congestive failure | Low | Irregular | Irregular | May be increased | Abnormal | Inconstant | Frequently shows improvement with digitalization |
| Rheumatic fever a. acute | Variable | May be irregular | May be indefinite | Normal in about one half | Abnormal | Not constant |  |
| b. chronic R.H.D. | Variable; high in aortic insufficiency | Usually regular; irregular in failure and sometimes in fibrillation | Usually definite | Usually normal | May get high N in mitral stenosis; H low to absent in fibrillation; K shallow in aortic stenosis | Constant | Presence of failure and/or arrhythmia will affect pattern |
| Coarctation of the aorta | Usually normal | Regular | Well defined | Normal | Deep I; shallow and slurred K; normal K sometimes | Constant | K may be shallow in normal children |
| Hypotension | Low to normal | Regular | Well defined | Normal | Shallow K-waves | Constant |  |
| Pulmonary disease | Usually normal | Often artifacts | Yes | Usually increased | Normal | Constant |  |
| Pericarditis | Variable; low in constrictive pericarditis | May be irregular | May be indefinite |  | Abnormal | Variable |  |

FIGURE 76.

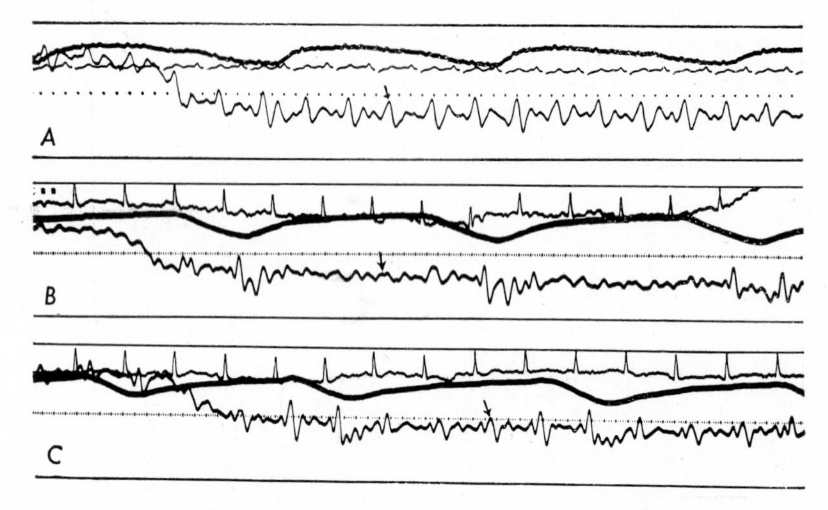


Sympathectomy—Reversal of Respiratory Variation with Binders

FIGURE 77. Three records of the same patient taken before (*A*) and after sympathectomy (*B* and *C*). (*A*) Ballistocardiograms of a hypertensive patient before dorsal sympathectomy. (*B*) Tracing of same patient as in *A* taken soon after a bilateral dorsal sympathectomy. Note the marked diminution in amplitude of the IJ stroke in expiration causing an increased (abnormal) respiratory variation. Compare expiratory beats in *A* with *B* (arrows). (*C*) Ballistocardiogram of same patient taken same day as in *B,* but after the application of abdominal and leg binders. Note the increased amplitude of the expiratory complexes (compare *B* and *C* arrows), and the more normal (decreased) respiratory variation. (deLalla, V., Jr., and Brown, H. R., Jr.: "The Respiratory Variation of the Ballistocardiogram," *Am. J. Med.,* **9**:728, 1950.)

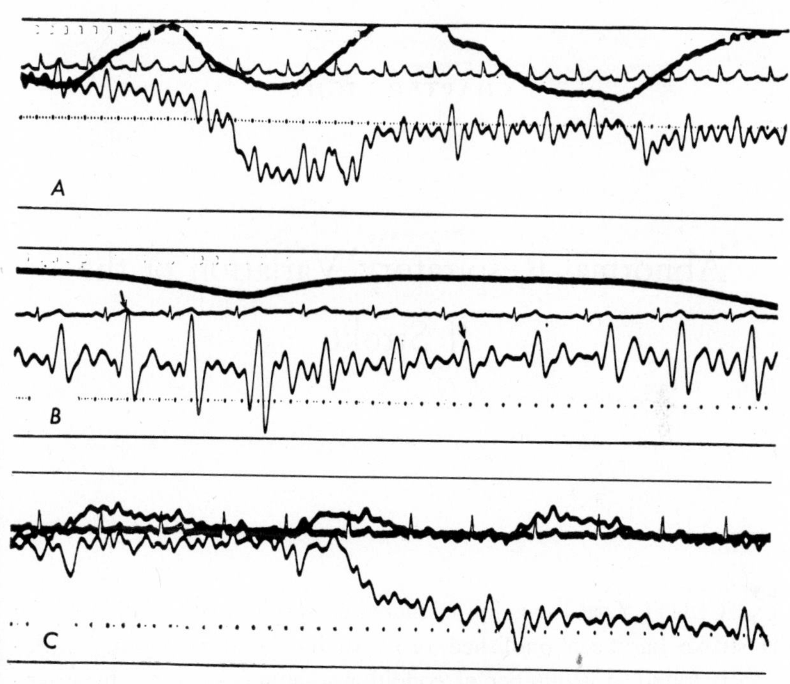


Emphysema and Fibrosis

FIGURE 78. Note the increased respiratory variation which is well shown in tracing *B*. (Compare first and second arrows.) (Trace *B* from de-Lalla, V., Jr., and Brown, H. R., Jr.: "The Respiratory Variation of the Ballistocardiogram," *Am. J. Med.*, **9**:728, 1950.)

CHAPTER EIGHT

# Abnormal Respiratory Variation of the IJ Stroke

RECENTLY, a discussion of increased respiratory variation of the IJ stroke has been published (*1*). An increased respiratory variation is found in a number of conditions—angina pectoris, hypertension, pulmonary emphysema, post bilateral sympathectomy cases, resistance breathing, and normals subjected to cold (*2*) (Figures 76, 77, and 78).

Normally, the amplitude of the IJ stroke diminishes slightly with expiration, as described in Chapter 6. This expiratory diminution is a reflection of the respiratory variation of the total ventricular output (algebraic sum of right and left ventricular stroke volumes), which also shows a slight decrease in expiration (*3* and *4*). It is our present belief that a normal respiratory variation depends partly upon the presence of a pulmonary pool as well as on normal function of the left and right ventricles. It seems evident that any situation which selectively damages the right ventricle or interferes with right ventricular output will tend to decrease the respiratory variation, i.e., allow the left ventricular variation to predominate. In the same fashion specific damage or interference with the left ventricle will increase the respiratory variation (allow the right ventricular variation to become even more predominant). This may be a possible explanation for the increased respiratory variation that is frequently seen post-infarction, since it is known that the majority of infarcts involve the left ventricle (*5*), it would also help to account for the increased respiratory variation seen in hypertensives, with or without failure, since that disease involves the left ventricle specifically.

However, we have certain evidence to show that an increased respiratory variation may also be caused by a diminution of the pulmonary pool. It has been shown by several observers that a pulmonary pool exists and that it is of considerable magnitude (*6, 7,* and *8*). The presence of this large pool of intravascular blood probably acts as a cushion between the right and left ventricles. Thus, it prevents the relatively drastic changes of the right heart output that occur with variations in intrapleural pressure from being transmitted to the systemic circulation via the left ventricle. This mechanism is augmented by the same intrathoracic respiratory pressure changes that cause the right heart variation: when the intrathoracic (intrapleural) pressure is increased by expiration, the venous return to the right heart is diminished, thereby decreasing the output, but the venous return to the left heart is enhanced, thereby increasing the left heart output at a time when the output of the right heart is diminished. The reverse occurs with inspiration; when the intrapleural pressure becomes more negative, the venous return increases to the right heart and decreases to the left heart (*3* and *4*).

The importance of these effects can be seen when one considers that the right heart output may frequently drop to critical levels during forced expirations, bouts of coughing, prolonged sighing, etc. If the cushioning effect of the pulmonary pool were not present, it is likely that syncope caused by cerebral anoxia would supervene, since the left ventricular output would also be seriously diminished. It is possible that this is the sequence of events in patients with tussive syncope where bouts of coughing may be of such a nature as to exhaust the pulmonary pool, or where the pulmonary pool is already critically low owing to other causes (Figure 79) (*1*).

It was the observation that a marked increase in the ballistocardiogram respiratory variation was produced in hypertensive patients subsequent to a bilateral dorsal sympathectomy that led to the experi-

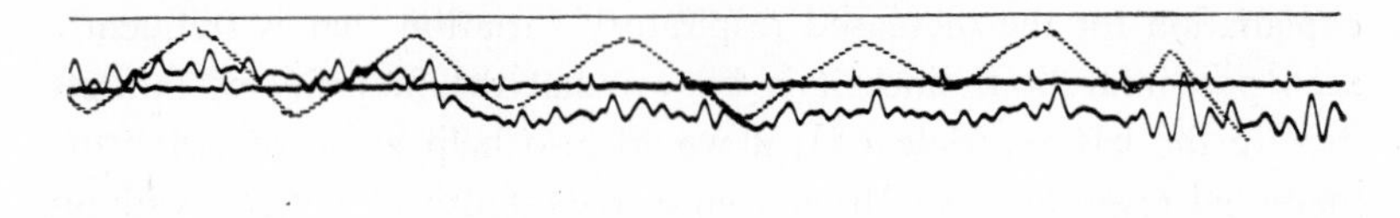

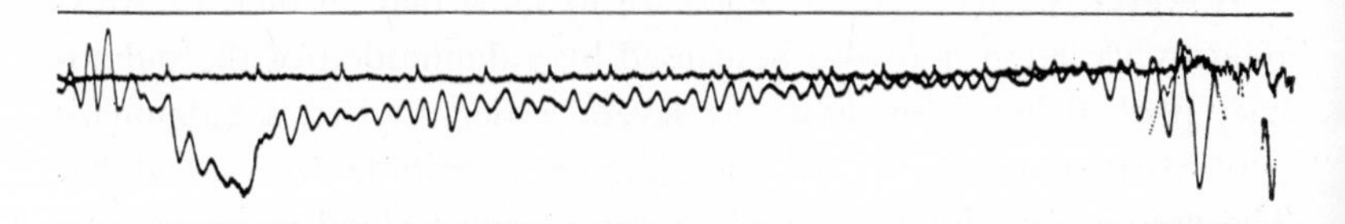

Tussive Syncope

FIGURE 79. Continuous record of a patient with tussive syncope taken just before and during a Valsalva maneuver. The onset of the Valsalva occurs at the beginning of the lower trace which is continuous with the upper record. Note the progressive diminution in amplitude as the Valsalva is held, finally ending in syncope and convulsions, occurring at the far right of the lower trace.

mental work presented below. Our interest was further stimulated by this same finding in patients with angina pectoris (*1* and *2*).

Destruction of the dorsal sympathetic chains results in pooling of large amounts of blood in the splanchnic region and the legs. This pooling diminishes the venous return to the right heart, so that many patients develop hypotension and syncope on standing. These post-sympathectomy individuals also show an increase in the ballistocardiogram respiratory variation, together with a very low expiratory amplitude of the IJ stroke (Figure 77, *B*). It is possible that the increased pooling in the splanchnic and leg areas decreases the pulmonary pool to such an extent that it no longer effectively cushions the respiratory changes of the right heart output, and therefore, the output of the left heart more nearly parallels that of the right. This would account for the observation that it is the expiratory beats which are abnormally low (Figure 77, *B*) since the right heart output diminishes with expiration. Under these circumstances the respiratory variation of the total output would more closely reflect the right heart respiratory variation, producing the changes observed in the ballistocardiogram.

Evidence for this was derived by taking ballistocardiograms on sympathectomized patients with and without supportive abdominal belt and stockings. Presumably, these binders prevent leg and splanchnic blood pooling to a large extent, and maintain the blood pressure above syncopal levels. This effect is illustrated by blood-pressure records taken on a patient, Mr. R., who experienced standing hypotension and syncope following a bilateral sympathectomy. His blood pressure was 200/110 lying down, but dropped to 80/65 within 4 min of passive standing. When he was placed in a rubber boot filled with water up to the iliac crests, he was able to stand passively for 15 min, and his blood pressure never fell below 120/80.

Figure 77 shows how the respiratory variation increased in a patient following bilateral dorsal sympathectomy (compare *A* with *B*). She developed hypotension and syncope when standing. When a tight abdominal binder and elastic stocking were applied, she was more comfortable, and she was able to stand for longer periods of time without syncope. A ballistocardiogram taken with these supports on showed that the respiratory variation had promptly decreased (approached normal) (compare *B* with *C* in Figure 77). Thus, the respiratory variation increased when the pulmonary pool diminished following bilateral sympathectomy and the subsequent splanchnic and leg pooling, and decreased when the pulmonary pool was increased, following application of binders.

Interestingly enough, an occasional postsympathectomy patient develops precordial chest pain on standing which is relieved by slight exertion, but especially relieved by lying down with the legs elevated. Presumably, the pain is derived from insufficient coronary blood flow owing to a very low left ventricular output. One such case was studied by us; the ballistocardiogram showed an abnormal pattern of very low amplitude. When an abdominal binder was applied the patient felt more comfortable, and the ballistocardiogram amplitude increased. This observation, which has already been reported (*1*), led to the study of the effects of an abdominal binder in patients with angina pectoris (see Chapter 11).

The possible causative relationship between a diminished pulmonary pool and coronary insufficiency is intriguing. It might be construed from the above that the pulmonary pool is diminished in those individuals who have coronary insufficiency with an increased ballistocardiogram respiratory variation. It is conceivable that in certain cases the primary cause of insufficient coronary blood flow is the diminished pulmonary blood pool which produces a critical diminution of the left ventricular output in expiration. During this period the disease process might be reversible. However, later it might be expected that an irreversible state would develop.

Since so many patients with coronary insufficiency complain of discomfort and pain in cold weather, it was considered of interest to determine the effect upon the ballistocardiogram of sudden exposure of the body to a cold environment. Accordingly, 5 normal male adults were rested upon the ballistocardiograph table, and, after control tracings had been taken, they were exposed to a room temperature of 60°F by quickly removing the blankets which had been covering them. Serial ballistocardiographic records were taken, together with blood pressures, up to the point of shivering. In all the cases the ballistocardiogram changed in a manner that increased the respiratory variation, producing a pattern much like that seen in coronary insufficiency and in resistance breathing (Figure 76). The increased respiratory variation noted might be due to a reflex producing either peripheral pooling of blood or to increased pulmonary resistance to breathing (see below), or to both.

A 51-year-old male who had been experiencing precordial pain for 18 months, and who complained of pain when subjected to cold, was similarly exposed to a room temperature of 60°F. His control tracings showed a low output, with an abnormal pattern and increased respiratory variation. Within 30 sec of exposure to the cold, his pattern had decreased in amplitude, indicating a still lower cardiac output, and his respiratory variation had increased. Within 1 min he began to experience precordial pain, and the experiment was discontinued. Upon warming, his pain diminished and then disappeared, and his tracing improved. Anxiety may have played a role in the production of pain. However, whatever the cause, there were an associated decrease in amplitude and increase in the respiratory variation of the ballistocardiogram.

An increased respiratory variation was also observed in patients with emphysema. This was interpreted as an exaggeration of the normal events produced by the increased respiratory intrapleural pressure variations that were present in these patients, i.e., increased negative pressures on inspiration and increased positive pressure on expiration (*10* and *11*). Thus, the effects of respiration on the venous return to both right and left heart would be exaggerated, and therefore the output variation would be greater. Also, since expiration (in time) usually occupies 60 to 70 per cent of the respiratory cycle in these patients, it might be deduced that the increased intrapulmonary positive pressure that is obtained in expiration would diminish the pulmonary pool just as positive-pressure breathing does (*7*).

This theory was partially confirmed by the work of Cain (*12*) who had 5 normal subjects breath through a resistance. He reported that the ballistocardiogram respiratory variation was increased immediately upon the start of resistance breathing which increased the alveolar pressure in expiration and decreased it in inspiration (see Figure 76).

A further attempt was made to determine whether any shift in pulmonary blood pool also occurred when breathing through a resistance. Accordingly, the same 5 subjects who showed an increased respiratory variation with resistance breathing were balanced on a teeterboard, using the method described by Fenn and co-workers (*7*). After a suitable base line had been obtained, the resistance was turned on. An immediate footward shift of weight occurred in each case. However, it is possible that the diaphragm shifts downward during resistance breathing and, in doing so, might have caused all of the footward shift observed. Therefore, one of the subjects, who was experienced and adept at controlling diaphragm movements, was allowed to hold a complete forced expiration several times during the control period, resistance-breathing period, and recovery period. By this means it was thought that the diaphragm would be fixed in a constant position, and its effect on the teeterboard would be eliminated during those brief periods of complete expiration. Comparison of the teeterboard levels during held expiration showed that a footward shift of weight had occurred with resistance breathing which presumably was independent of the position of the diaphragm (Figure 80). This footward shift may be interpreted to mean that during resistance breathing blood is driven out of the pulmonary pool, and

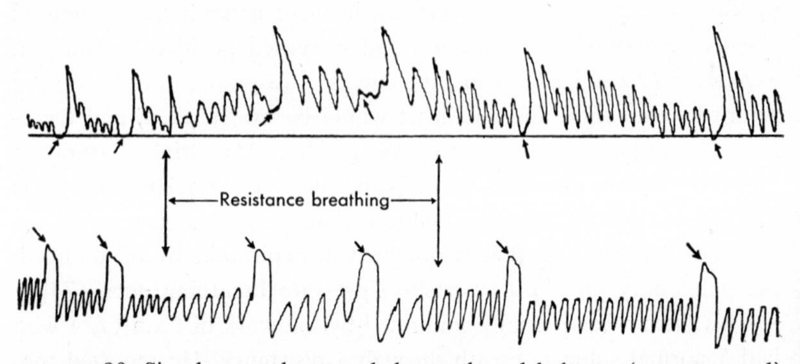


FIGURE 80. Simultaneously recorded teeterboard balance (upper record) and respirations (lower record expiration upon a normal male adult before, during, and after resistance breathing). The large undulations of the teeterboard balance are caused by the movement of the diaphragm with respiration: the footward (down on tracing) inspiratory movement of the diaphragm causes a footward shift of weight of the teeterboard (upward deflection). The arrows point to held forced expirations; note that the teeterboard undulations stop, and the pointer writes a relatively straight line. This short base line reflects the distribution of blood. Note that during resistance breathing the teeterboard becomes foot heavy (upward deflection), and that the expiratory base lines (arrows) remain higher than either the control or recovery periods even though the diaphragm presumably occupied the same position in all cases. This is taken to mean that resistance breathing caused a shift of blood in a footward direction (see text). (deLalla, V., Jr., and Brown, H. R., Jr.: "The Respiratory Variation of the Ballistocardiogram," *Am. J. Med.,* **9**:728, 1950.)

that most of it is taken up by the splanchnic and leg pools. Therefore, it seems reasonable to assume that during resistance breathing a diminution of the pulmonary blood pool occurred at the same time that the ballistocardiogram respiratory variation increased.

Upon the basis of the above series of experiments, it might be deduced that an increased respiratory variation may very likely be associated with a diminution in the pulmonary blood pool in certain conditions; from the evidence at hand it seems to be caused by this diminution as well as by left ventricular damage. The decrease in the pulmonary pool could be caused either by increased intrapulmonary pressure on expiration, such as occurs during resistance breathing, or by an increase in the peripheral and splanchnic blood pools, such as occurs following a bilateral dorsal sympathectomy. It is also possible that, in certain cases at least, coronary insufficiency might be secondary to a critically low left ventricular output caused by increased peripheral pooling and a consequent decreased pulmonary pool.

## REFERENCES

### ABNORMAL RVI SECTION

1. deLalla, V., Jr., and Brown, H. R., Jr.: "The Respiratory Variation of the Ballistocardiogram," *Am. J. Med.,* **9**:728, 1950.
2. Brown, H. R., Jr., and deLalla, V., Jr.: "The Ballistocardiogram, Description and Clinical Use," *Am. J. Med.,* **9**:718, 1950.
3. Boyd, T. C., and Patras, M.: "Variations in Filling and Output of Ventricles with Phases of Respiration," *Am. J. Physiol.,* **134**:75, 1941.
4. Shuler, R., Ensor, C., Gunning, R., Moss, W., and Johnson, V.: "Differential Effects of Respiration on Left and Right Ventricles," *Am. J. Physiol.,* **137**:602, 1942.
5. Barnes, A. R., and Ball, R. G.: "The Incidence and Situation of Myocardial Infarction in One Thousand Consecutive Post-Mortem Examinations," *Am. J. M. Sc.,* **183**:215, 1932.
6. Best, C. H., and Taylor, N. B.: "The Physiological Basis of Medical Practice," Wm. Wood and Co., Baltimore, Md., **4**:283, 1945.
7. Fenn, W., Otis, A., Rahn, H., Chadwick, L., and Hegnauer, A.: "Displacement of Blood from the Lungs by Pressure Breathing," *Am. J. Physiol.,* **151**:258, 1947.
8. Visscher, M. B.: "Capacity Changes in Pulmonary Vascular Bed with Respiratory Cycle," *Federation Proc.,* **7**:128, 1948.
9. Brown, H. R., Jr., Hoffman, M. J., and deLalla, V., Jr.: "Ballistocardiographic Findings in Patients with Symptoms of Angina Pectoris," *Circulation,* **1**:132, 1950.
10. Paine, J. R.: "Clinical Measurement of Pulmonary Elasticity," *J. Thoracic Surg.,* **9**:550, 1940.
11. Dean, R. B., and Visscher, M. B.: "The Kinetics of Lung Ventilation," *Am. J. Physiol.,* **134**:450, 1941.
12. Cain, C. C., and Otis, A. B.: "Some Physiological Effects Resulting from Added Resistance to Respiration," *J. Aviation Med.,* **20**:149, 1949.

**CHAPTER NINE**

# Hypertension

---

THE ballistocardiogram will never replace the blood-pressure cuff in the diagnosis of hypertension; however, it does add information concerning the status of the heart and its function under the continued stress of systemic hypertension.

Perhaps the first change that occurs in the ballistocardiogram pattern with hypertension is a deepening of the K-wave (Figure 81, *A* and *B*). This is in keeping with the theory that the K-wave is produced by deceleration of the impulse wave in the legs by peripheral resistance. In early stages the output may be normal, and the respiratory variation may be normal (Figure 81, *B*). At some time in the progress of the disease the respiratory variation increases, and the cardiac output decreases (Figure 81, *C* and *D*). These changes may be entirely related to peripheral or pulmonary vascular phenomena, abnormal blood pooling for instance, or may involve changes in muscular efficiency of the left ventricle. Still later in the disease process, however, there appear marked changes in the over-all pattern—shallow I valley, high IJ take-off, and a pronounced expiratory diminution in amplitude of the IJ stroke, indicating impaired mechanical efficiency and probably low output (Figure 82). Patients with this sort of pattern have other evidence of hypertensive heart disease, frequently with a history of paroxysmal dyspnea, angina, or episodes of congestive failure.

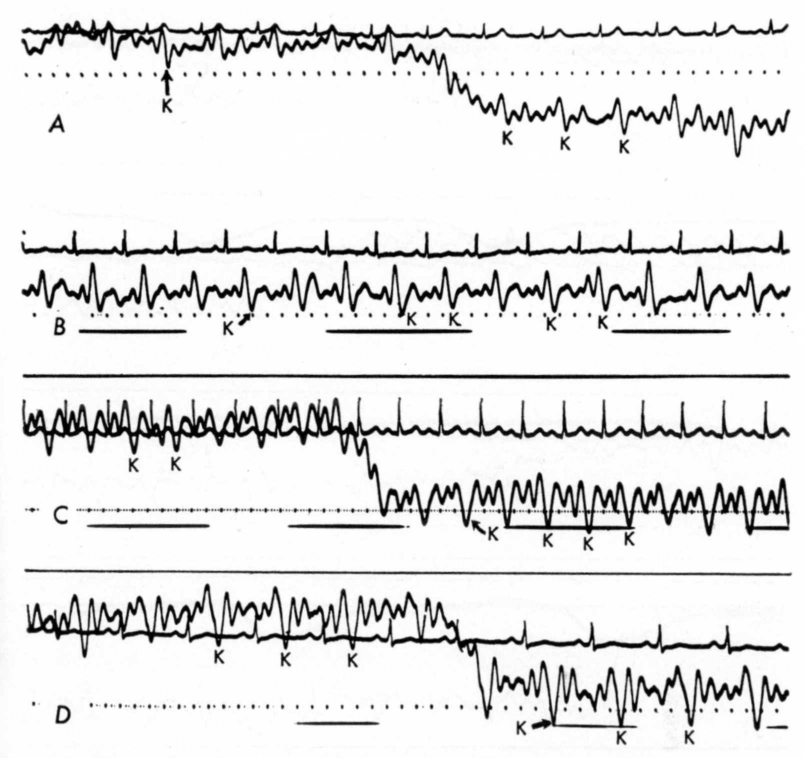


FIGURE 81. Four records of hypertensive patients. *A* and *B* show deep K-waves and increased respiratory variation. *C* and *D* showed a marked increase in the K valley, with low amplitude of complexes.

The deepening of the K-wave of the ballistocardiogram in hypertension is probably due to increased peripheral resistance, together with increased rigidity of arterial and arteriolar walls. Qualitatively, this change is evaluated by comparing the depth of the I-wave to that of the K-wave. A quantitative index of this relationship is the JK/IJ ratio. This ratio is normally about 1, and it becomes considerably increased when the K-wave is abnormally deep.

In a few "normal" individuals the K-waves are deeper than usual, with a ratio of 1.3:1.5. Further investigation may possibly reveal that such subjects are prehypertensives or have arteriosclerosis. We cannot at present say that such is the case; nothing more can be said

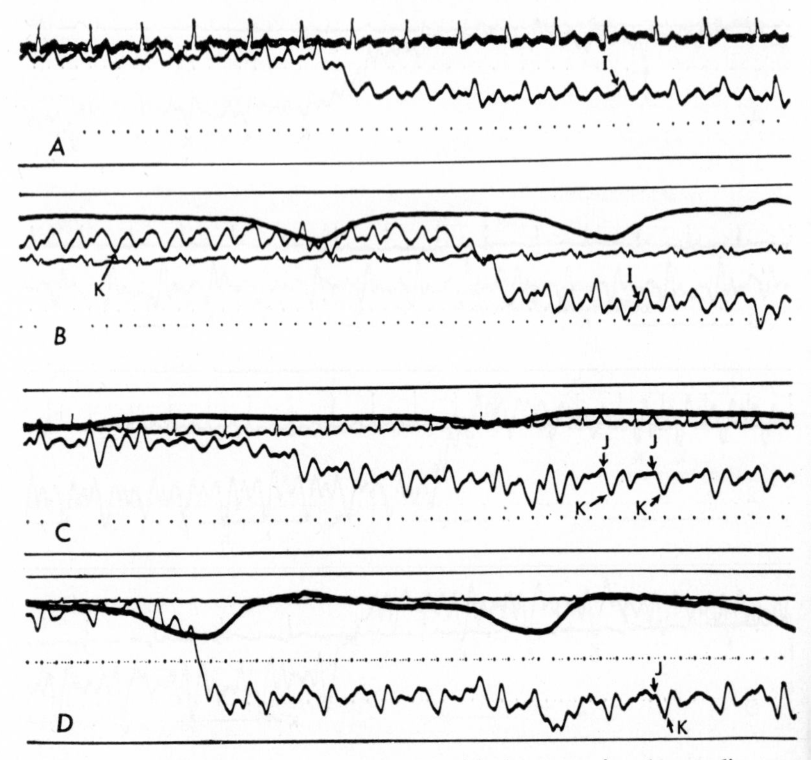


FIGURE 82. Records of four patients with hypertensive heart disease. These patterns are characterized by very low amplitude, shallow I valley, low IJ stroke [particularly in expiration (arrows)], and deep K-waves.

about deep K-waves in a normal subject except that the observation has been made, and no prognostic significance should be attached to this finding. Five in our series of "normals" were found to have a diastolic pressure of 90 or more. One of these subjects showed slightly deep K-waves, and the rest had normal tracings. A few others of our normal series had records with slightly deep K-waves. It can be seen that it is important that each patient's blood pressure be taken before and after the tracing. Every patient should be allowed to rest on the table for at least 10 min; in order to evaluate changes with rest, it is desirable to take a record as soon as the subject lies down and again after 10 to 15 min rest.

The K-wave deepens in hypertension, but no threshold for this change has been established. It can be stated that with a blood pressure of 180/110 or more, the K-waves are usually deep. Other variables, such as the rigidity of the vessel walls, are contributing factors, and more specific limits cannot be set. Figure 83 shows an example

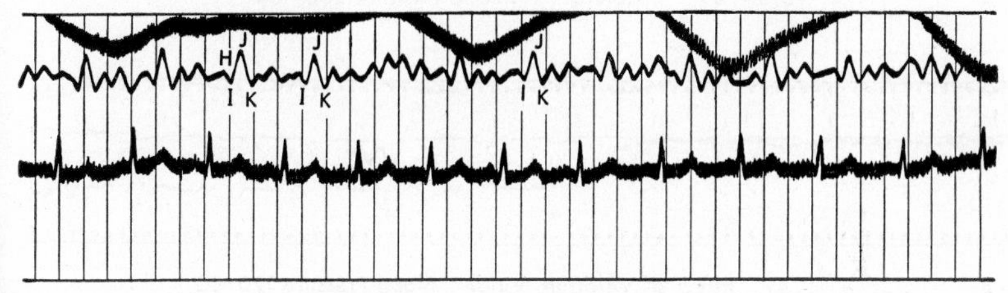


Hypertension Normal K-Wave

FIGURE 83. A record taken on a 7-year-old girl whose blood pressure was 160/120; note the normal K-waves. This is probably because the soft arterial walls dampened out the arterial pulse.

of this variability—it is a record on a 7-year-old girl with a blood pressure of 160/120, and the pattern is entirely normal, probably because the soft arterial walls that are found in children dampen out the force of the impulse wave. Coarctation of the aorta should be suspected when a patient with a marked brachial hypertension shows beats with comparatively shallow K-waves.

We have observed changes in the K-wave with lowering of blood pressure in two circumstances: (1) treatment with veratrum viride, and (2) postsympathectomy patients. In 2 patients treated with veratrum viride decreased blood pressure and a simultaneous decrease in the K valley were seen. Figure 84 shows traces taken before and during veratrum viride treatment in such a situation. In 2 other patients veratrum viride produced little change in either the blood pressure or the K-wave.

Immediately after sympathectomy the pattern may become even more abnormal, usually with an increased respiratory variation and a decreased amplitude. This was also the observation of Starr (*3*) (Figures 85 and 86). This phenomenon is thought to be due to the increased peripheral pooling (splanchnic and legs) that occurs (*1* and

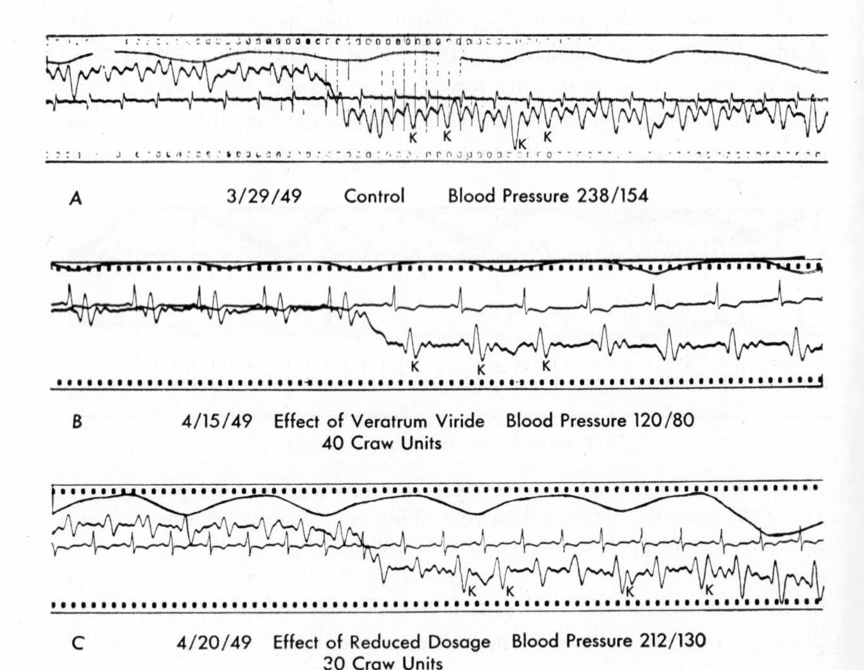


FIGURE 84. Records taken from a hypertensive woman before and during veratrum viride treatment. Note the normal-appearing pattern in *B* when the blood pressure was lowered to normal limits. The K-waves become less deep when the tension is lowered and become deeper again in *C* when the blood pressure rises.

*2*); many of these patients also have postural standing hypotension. An abdominal support to decrease splanchnic pooling and aid venous return will result in improvement clinically as well as in the ballistocardiogram (Figure 85) (*1* and *2*).

Several months after sympathectomy, presumably after a certain amount of vessel tone has been re-established, the pattern amplitude may increase, and the respiratory variation and K-wave may approach normal (Figure 86).

No long-term, carefully planned ballistocardiographic studies of hypertensives are available. Starr has reported that the ballistocardiogram is of low amplitude in hypertensives with small hearts and of

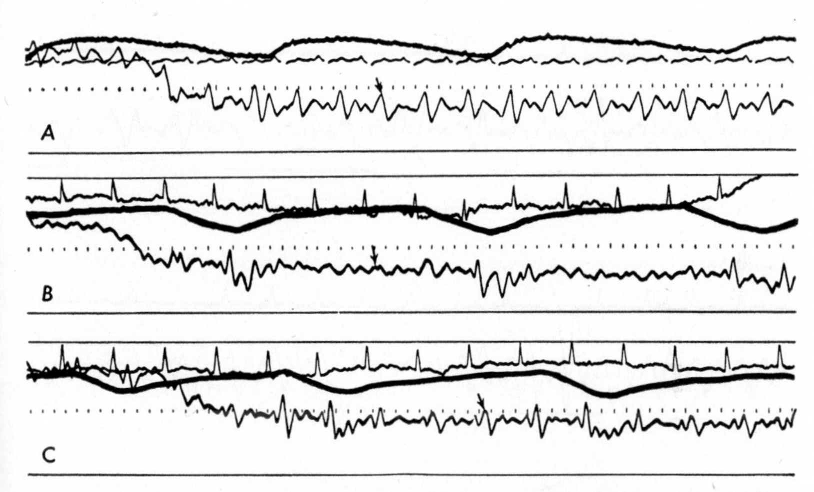


Sympathectomy—Reversal of Respiratory Variations with Binders

FIGURE 85. Three records taken on a hypertensive patient before (*A*) and 2 weeks after (*B* and *C*) a dorsal sympathectomy. Tracing *B* was taken without abdominal binders or elastic stockings. Note the marked decrease of amplitude of the expiratory patterns (arrow) as compared with *A* and the consequent increase of respiratory variation. Tracing *C* was taken immediately after tracing *B*, but with a rigid abdominal support and elastic stockings applied. Note the increase in the amplitude of the expiratory beats (arrow) as compared with *B*. The sensitivity of the ballistocardiograph amplifier was kept constant for tracings *B* and *C*. (Brown, H. R., Jr., and deLalla, V., Jr.: "The Ballistocardiogram, Description and Clinical Use," *Am. J. Med.*, **9**:718, 1950.)

larger amplitude in hypertensives with large hearts (*4* and *5*). It can be said that, generally, deterioration of the ballistocardiogram toward an irregular, indefinite, low-amplitude record goes along with progression of the disease (Figure 82). This probably indicates impaired mechanical heart action secondary to hypertension or coronary involvement, or both. The ballistocardiogram gives a fairly good index of the degree of myocardial damage or "strain" present in hypertensive patients.

In our laboratory over the past 2 years, a total of 230 patients with hypertension have been studied with the ballistocardiogram. Of these, 5 had normal records and 10 had borderline tracings; 52 were

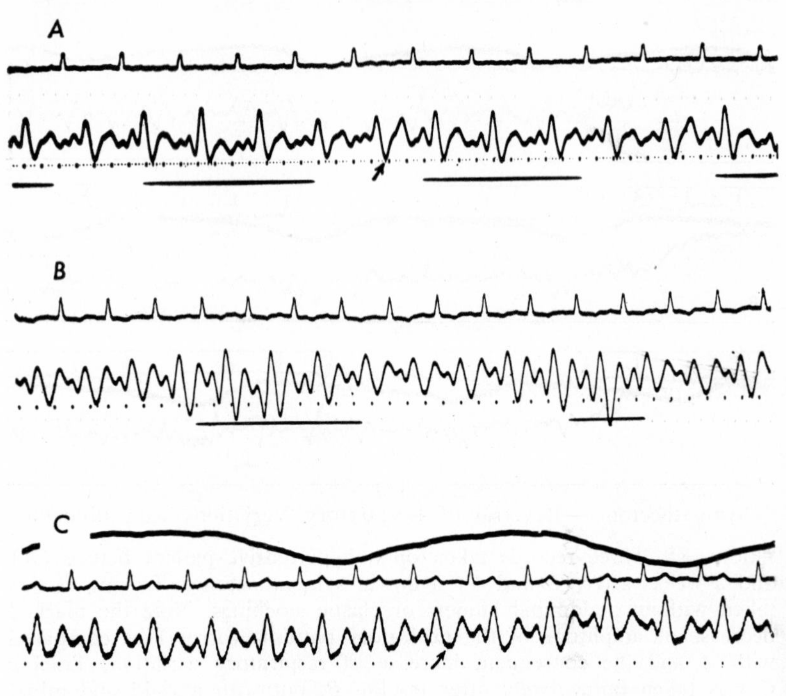


FIGURE 86. Three records taken on a hypertensive patient before and after bilateral dorsal sympathectomy. (*A*) Tracing taken before operation, blood pressure 240/120. Note the characteristic deep K-wave (arrow) and the increased respiratory variation. (*B*) Tracing taken 2 weeks following the second stage of operation. Note the increased respiratory variation. (*C*) Tracing taken 3 months later when the blood pressure was 130/80. Note the more shallow and slurred K-waves and the normal respiratory variation.

slightly abnormal; 115 were moderately abnormal; 48 had markedly abnormal records.

Of this group, 38 underwent a bilateral dorsal sympathectomy. These findings are summarized in Figure 87, *A*. This may not be a true representation of the relationship of the ballistocardiogram to hypertensives considered suitable for sympathectomy, since the series is relatively small. Also, ballistocardiograms were requested more frequently on candidates for operation than on those who were not considered suitable. Because of the small number of operated patients, long-term ballistocardiogram changes postoperatively cannot be presented.

| *Type of Ballistocardiogram Pattern* | *Number of Patients* | *Number Operated* | *Per Cent of Operated Patients* |
|---|---|---|---|
| Normal | 5 | 0 | |
| Borderline | 10 | 0 | |
| Slightly abnormal | 52 | 9 | 23.7 |
| Moderately abnormal | 115 | 22 | 58.0 |
| Markedly abnormal | 48 | 7 | 18.3 |
| Total | 230 | 38 | |

A. *Relation of Type of Pattern to Per Cent Hypertensives Operated*

| *Ballistocardiogram Pattern* | *Subjects* | | *Patients with Coronary Disease* | | *Patients with Hypertensive Heart Disease* | |
|---|---|---|---|---|---|---|
| | *Number* | *Per Cent* | *Number* | *Per Cent* | *Number* | *Per Cent* |
| Slightly abnormal | 52 | 25.5 | 4 | 10.5 | 0 | 0 |
| Moderately abnormal | 115 | 52.1 | 17 | 44.75 | 14 | 61 |
| Markedly abnormal | 48 | 22.4 | 17 | 44.75 | 9 | 39 |
| Total | 215 | | 38 | | 23 | |

B. *Relation of Type of Pattern to Per Cent Hypertensives with Heart Disease*

FIGURE 87

Generally, the ballistocardiogram pattern shows a more marked abnormality in those who have angina pectoris, a previous coronary occlusion, or hypertensive heart disease. This relationship is shown in Figure 87, *B*. Starr has shown that hypertensives in failure may show a fairly regular, high-amplitude pattern (Figure 88).

In summary, the ballistocardiogram usually shows changes in early, mild hypertension as well as in advanced cases. The K-wave changes are relatively specific, and with progression of the disease more nonspecific effects of myocardial damage or coronary disease are seen. Treatment, both medical and surgical, can be evaluated with the ballistocardiogram provided that controls are adequate. The presence of myocardial involvement or coronary disease may be confirmed with the help of the ballistocardiogram.

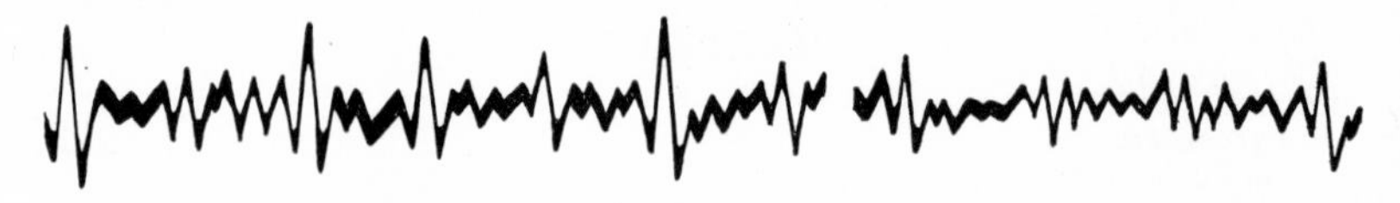


FIGURE 88. Figure showing a high-amplitude (high-output) pattern in a hypertensive in congestive failure. Note the reduction in amplitude following digitalization. This is not the usual result of digitalis in congestive failure (see Chapter 13). (Starr, I.: "Clinical Studies with the Ballistocardiograph," *Am. J. M. Sc.,* **202**:469, 1941.)

# REFERENCES

## HYPERTENSION

1. deLalla, V., Jr., and Brown, R. H., Jr.: "The Respiratory Variation of the Ballistocardiogram," *Am. J. Med.,* **9**:728, 1950.
2. Brown, H. R., Jr., and deLalla, V., Jr.: "The Ballistocardiogram, Description and Clinical Use, *Am. J. Med.,* **9**:718, 1950.
3. Starr, I.: "Clinical Studies with the Ballistocardiograph," *Am. J. M. Sc.,* **202**:469, 1941.
4. Starr, I.: "On the Clinical Characteristics of Patients with Subnormal Circulation in the Absence of Acute Heart Failure," *Tr. A. Am. Physicians,* **54**:163, 1939.
5. Starr, I., and Jonas, L.: "Syndrome of Subnormal Circulation in Ambulatory Patients," *Arch. Int. Med.,* **66**:1095, 1940.

CHAPTER TEN

# Myocardial Infarction

THE ballistocardiographic abnormalities following myocardial infarction vary and may include any or all of the following, depending upon the degree of involvement. (1) *Increased respiratory variation:* this finding probably occurs in most post-infarction traces, but it may be obscured by other changes in amplitude and regularity. (2) *Irregular and indefinite patterns:* this type of abnormality may never occur; in patients where it is present and who survive, it may be seen from 1 to 10 days following infarction (presumably depending upon amount of muscle involved). When a large series is obtained it is to be expected that those individuals who have sustained a massive infarct will immediately show irregular and indefinite patterns. (3) *Decrease in amplitude:* this is particularly true in the case of the IJ stroke; it reflects a decreased cardiac output, and again, the degree of diminution will be a function of the amount of muscle involvement. Starr (*1*), in a series of 10 patients, demonstrated a progressive decrease of cardiac output in 7, reaching a minimum in 3 to 5 weeks. (4) *M-shaped waves:* these are frequently seen in patients after infarction, and they may persist indefinitely. These are characterized by low I-J-waves and high H- and L-waves. The significance of this is unknown, although Starr (*2*) produced similar patterns in dogs (Figure 89) following the application of a hot soldering iron to the wall of the right ventricle. He attributed this pattern to inequality

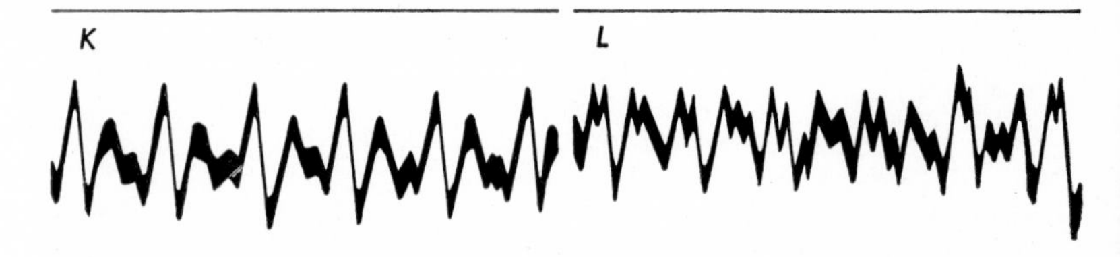


FIGURE 89. *K* is the ballistocardiogram pattern of a normal dog whose heart is surgically exposed. *L* is the pattern obtained following searing of the right ventricular wall with a red-hot iron. (Starr, I., Rawson, A. J., Schroeder, H. A., and Joseph, N. R.: "Studies on the Estimation of Cardiac Output in Man, and of Abnormalities in Cardiac Function, from the Heart's Recoil and the Blood's Impact; the Ballistocardiogram," *Am. J. Physiol.,* **127**:1, 1939.)

of ventricular function. We have seen M-shaped waves occur as early as 16 days following infarction in humans.

At this time it cannot be said with certainty exactly when the ballistocardiogram becomes abnormal following myocardial infarction because of lack of observations shortly before and immediately after infarction. The difficulty in obtaining an extensive number of serial traces lies in the undesirability of moving such patients from their bed to the ballistocardiograph table. This problem may be surmounted by portable direct recording apparatus similar to that described by Dock and Taubman (*3*).

It is conceivable that an infarct could be so minimal that there is no impairment of myocardial function and therefore no demonstrable abnormality of the ballistocardiogram at any time. However, in our series of over 55 patients, we have never seen a completely normal trace after infarction.

Five patients with myocardial infarction were followed with daily serial tracings, for periods up to 7 weeks. In one of these a record was obtained 36 hr after the attack; in the other four, the first tracing was taken 9 to 11 days after the attack. All patients showed an abnormal pattern at the time of the first trace; three out of five initial records showed irregular patterns, including the 36-hr trace. All of the initial patterns showed an increased respiratory variation, as exemplified by Figure 90, *A*. Four of the five initial patterns showed decreased amplitude, as exemplified by Figure 90, *B*.

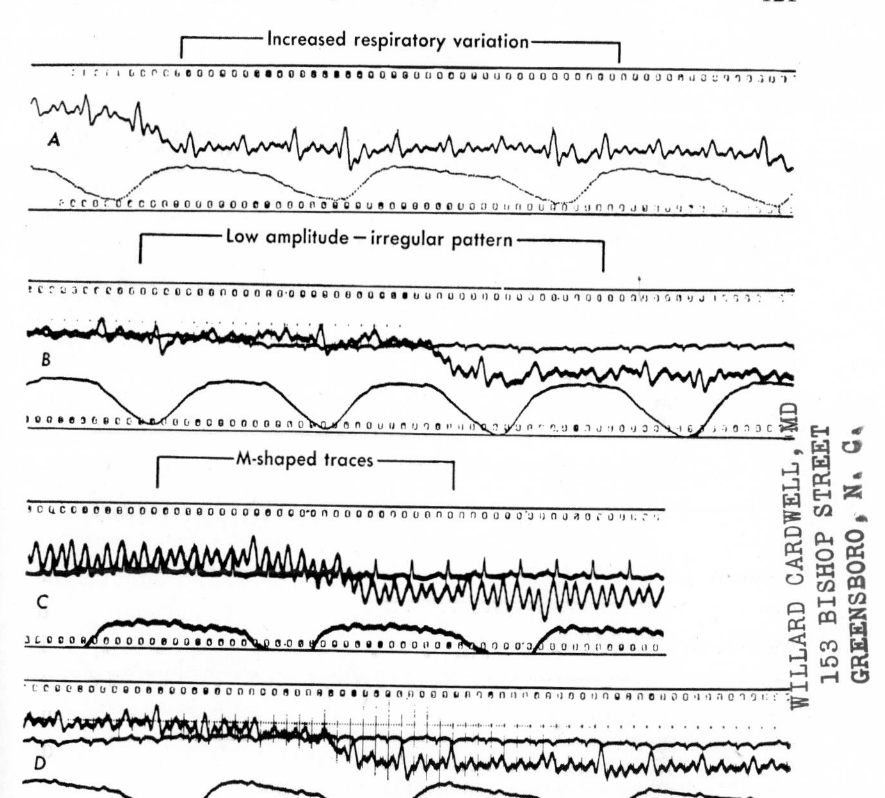




FIGURE 90. Records taken from patients with acute myocardial infarction. *A* was taken on a patient 9 days after infarction. *B* was taken 2½ days after infarction. *C* and *D* were taken 21 and 30 days post-infarction, respectively.

M-shaped patterns appeared in two of the group, one on the twenty-first day and another on the thirtieth day following infarction (Figure 90, *C* and *D*. Two of the cases showed improvement, in their ballistocardiograms and clinically (Figure 91), one in a 6 weeks' period and one after 8 weeks; two showed no change (Figure 92). Two of the series died, one of them 10 days following our last trace and the other 8 weeks following his infarction and after discharge from the hospital. Post-mortem findings confirmed the diagnosis in

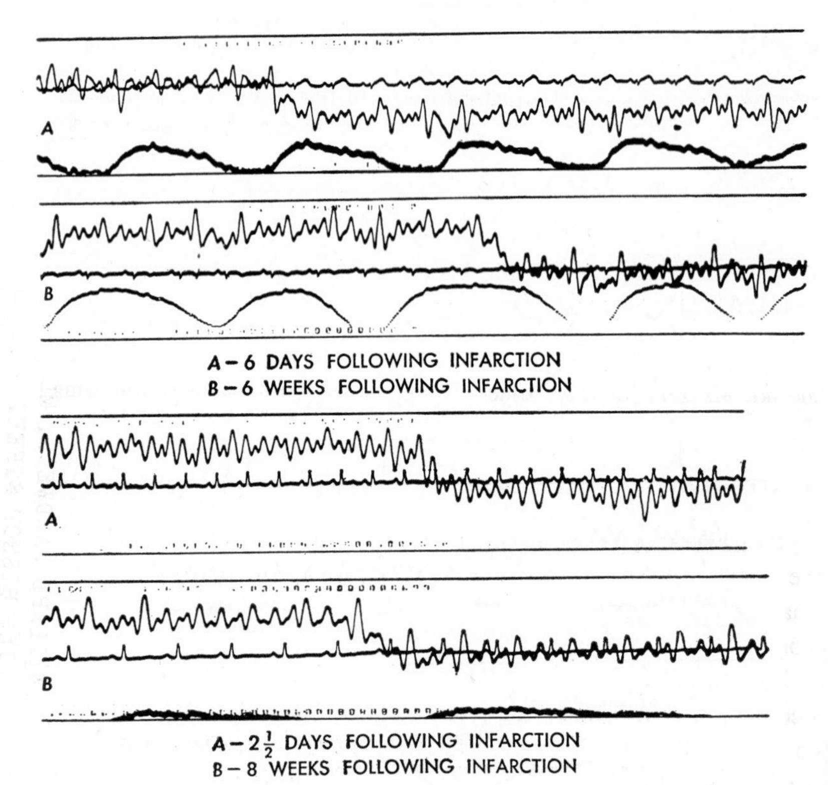


Traces Showing Improvement following Rest Periods after Myocardial Infarction

FIGURE 91. Compare *A* and *B* in both cases. Note the increased amplitude and regularity of the *B* records as contrasted with the *A* records.

one of the cases; a post-mortem examination was not performed in the other case.

We have obtained records on over 50 other patients who had sustained a myocardial infarction. All of these records are abnormal: 5 of the records were taken in the first month post-infarction; 5 were in the 1- to 6-month period; 5 in the 6- to 12-month period; and 35 were taken 1 year or more after the attack. Although all patterns were abnormal, only 10 were classified as very abnormal (Grade 4), with totally irregular patterns. This suggests that the prognosis is poor

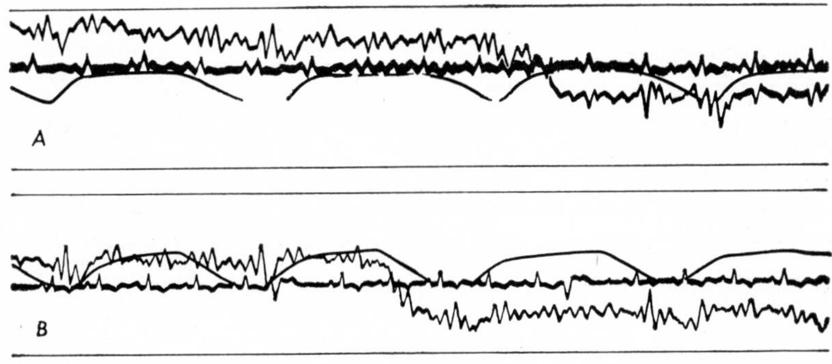


FIGURE 92. (*A*) 11 days following infarction; (*B*) 24 days following infarction.

in patients where this type of pattern persists. Forty-four traces were classified as moderately abnormal (Grades 2 and 3), with low amplitude, M-shaped waves, and abnormal respiratory variation. Six were classified as only slightly abnormal (Grade 1), with minimal changes in pattern or amplitude, or with increased respiratory variation.

Figures 93, 94, and 95 show the deterioration of pattern that may occur in the first weeks following infarction. Figure 95 shows changes in regularity, definitiveness, and amplitude of complexes that occurred in a period of 5 days following extension of a myocardial infarct in this patient.

Figure 96 shows the variations one may see in patterns one to several years following known coronary occlusion. Tracing 96, *A*, shows a nearly normal pattern of a patient who had his coronary attack in 1940. Serial yearly traces on this individual over the past 3 years have shown no variation from the trace portrayed here. Similarly, he has had no symptomatic complaints referable to his cardiovascular system, although he exercises great caution in all his activities. Tracing 96, *B*, is a record of a 61-year-old man following coronary occlusion. The low amplitude with low I-J-waves and high H- and L-waves give the complexes an M-shaped appearance which is a frequent ballistocardiogram finding in many of the old coronary occlusion cases. This pattern may be first seen at any time post-occlusion and may persist indefinitely. It is to be noted that M-shaped

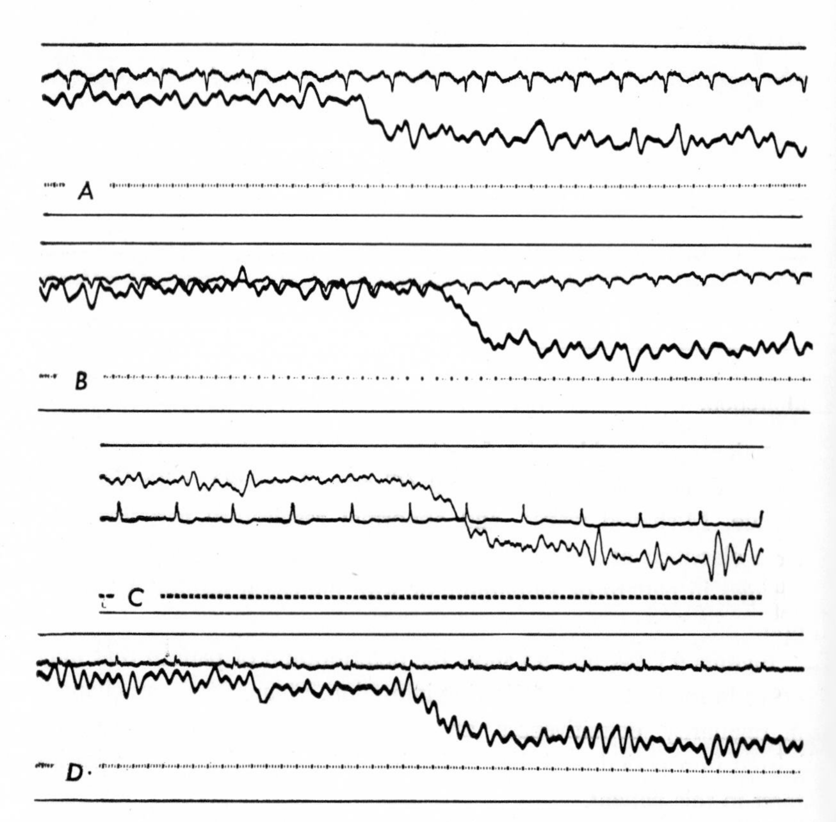


FIGURE 93. No respirations record. (*A*) A 49-year-old male with an anterior coronary occlusion one day old. Note the low amplitude and the irregularity of the complexes. (*B*) Same patient as in *A*, 45 days later. The output is very low and the complexes have become more irregular and indefinite. This indicates poor myocardial recovery. (*C*) An 82-year-old female two weeks after a posterior coronary occlusion. Note the very low output, and irregularity and indefiniteness of the pattern. (*D*) Same patient as in *C*, four weeks after occlusion. The record remains irregular and indefinite, but shows some improvement in amplitude.

beats are more prominent during expiration, owing to the shortened IJ stroke during that phase of respiration.

Figure 97 shows a series of patients, varying in ages from 52 to

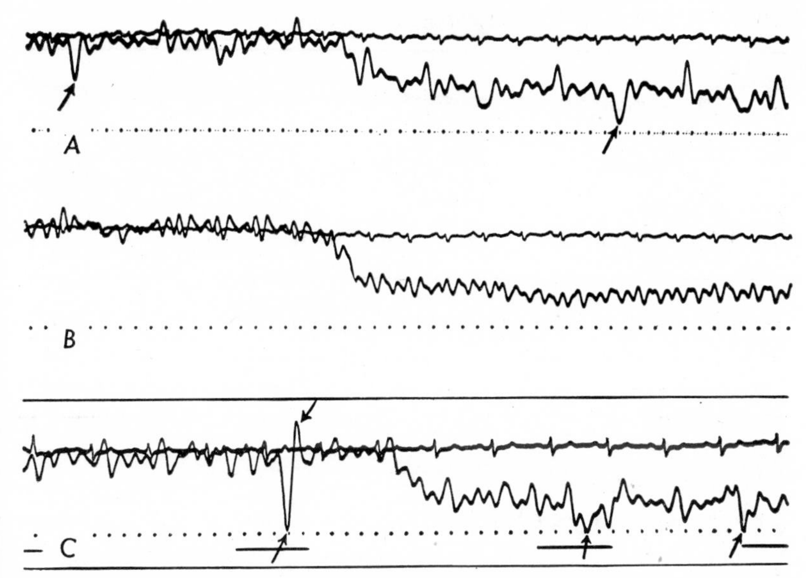


FIGURE 94. (*A*) A 62-year-old man 4 weeks after anterior coronary occlusion. The amplitude is low, and the complexes are irregular and indefinite. (*B*) Same patient 6 weeks following occlusion. Pattern is lower in amplitude, irregular, and indefinite, indicating poor recovery. (*C*) A 55-year-old man 6 weeks after a posterior occlusion. Note artefacts produced by motion of subject (arrows).

64, who are having moderately severe symptoms of angina pectoris following their myocardial infarctions 1 year previously. Note the irregular and indefinite complexes in *A,* the respiratory variations in *B* and *C,* and the M-shaped-appearance complexes in *D.*

Figure 98 is taken from Starr and shows progressive decline in amplitude of the ballistocardiogram pattern following myocardial infarction.

It can be seen that the ballistocardiogram is of help in the diagnosis of myocardial infarction, but that it is more useful in determining the status of the ventricular muscle post-infarction and in evaluating the amount of recovery that has occurred. In this respect it is perhaps of more value than the electrocardiogram, whereas the electrocardiogram remains paramount in diagnosis of the acute attack.

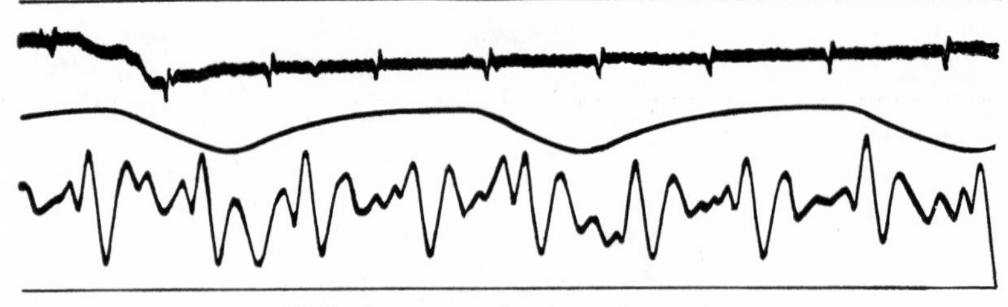

9/3/49 — 1 Day After Second Attack of
Tachycardia and Chest Pain

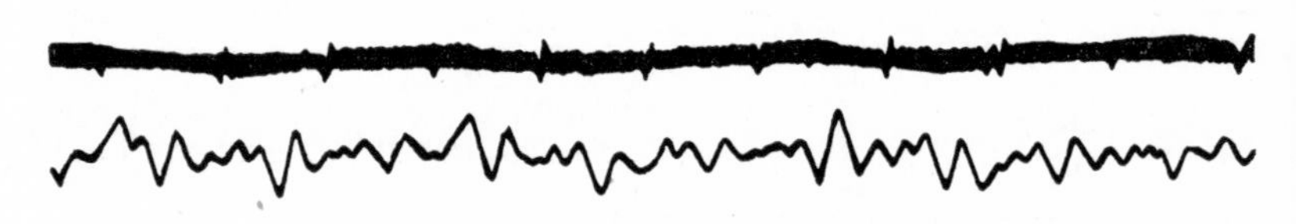

9/8/49 — Persistent Substernal Pain

FIGURE 95. This figure shows traces of a 31-year-old man who suffered an anterior myocardial infarction Sept. 1, 1948. The first ballistocardiogram was obtained in this laboratory Sept. 11, 1948. He returned to the hospital almost a year later, on Sept. 3, 1949, with severe chest pain, and the record obtained then, although abnormal in type, showed good regularity and definitiveness of complexes. The pain persisted, although the electrocardiogram, WBC, and sedimentation rate were entirely unremarkable. The pattern of Sept. 8, 1949, shows marked reduction in amplitude of the waves, with irregular and indefinite complexes.

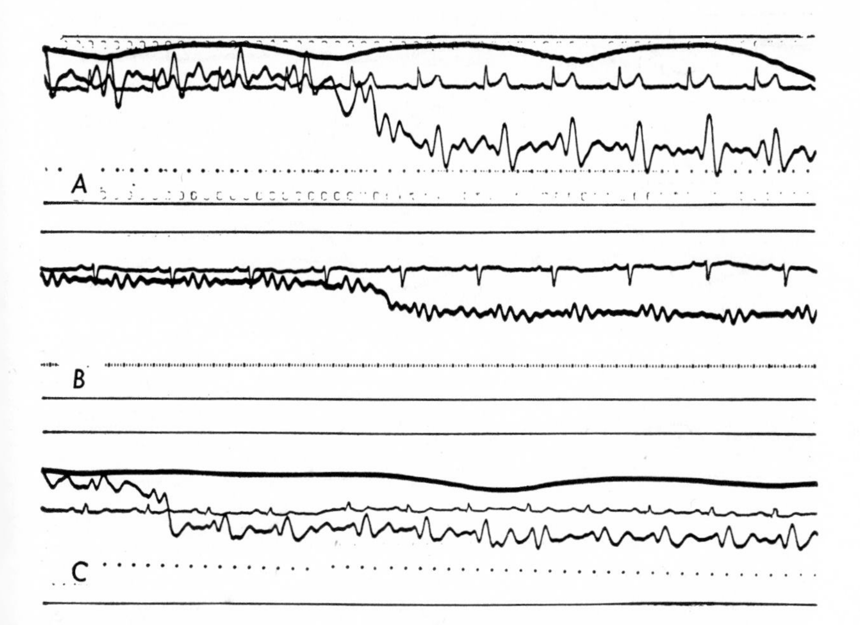


FIGURE 96. Records of three patients who have made a good recovery following myocardial infarction. (*A*) A 55-year-old male with history of coronary occlusion 10 years earlier. He has no pain. Note the normal amplitude, regularity, and definitiveness of pattern. This indicates an excellent recovery, with little impairment of muscular function. (*B*) A 61-year-old male who had a coronary occlusion 1 year ago. He has no pain. The output is low, but the pattern is regular and definite, and is abnormal by virtue of the high L peak, giving the complexes an M-shaped appearance. (*C*) A 66-year-old male with a 1-year-old coronary occlusion, who has no pain. Note the regularity and definitiveness of pattern. It is classed as abnormal because of the low output and the slurred K-wave. (Trace *A* from Brown, H. R., Jr., and deLalla, V., Jr.: "The Ballistocardiogram, Description and Clinical Use," *Am. J. Med.,* **9**:718, 1950.)

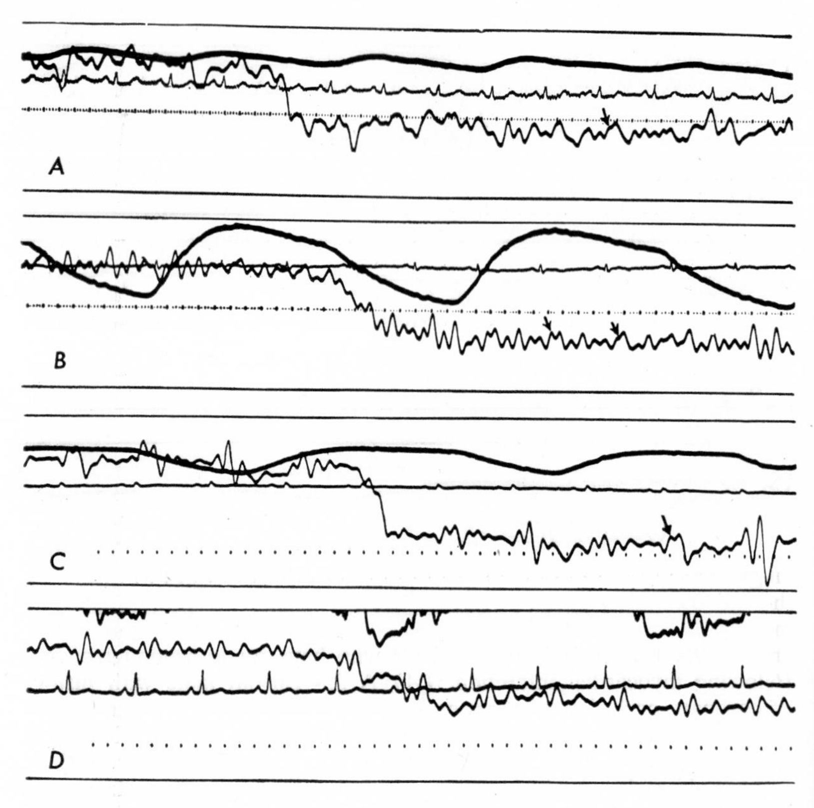


FIGURE 97. Records of four patients who have made a poor recovery following myocardial infarction. (*A*) A 52-year-old woman who had an occlusion 1 year prior. At the time of the tracing she complained of chest pain. The low amplitude and irregular, indefinite complexes indicate a poorly functioning myocardium. Note the expiratory beat pattern (arrow). (*B*) A 64-year-old male with a 1-year-old coronary occlusion, complaining of precordial pain. Note the high H, shallow I, and very high IJ take-off occurring in expiration (arrows), with an increased respiratory variation. (*C*) A 60-year-old male with a 1-year-old coronary occlusion, complaining of chest pain. Note the similarity of the expiratory beats to *B* (arrow). (*D*) A 55-year-old female with a 1-year-old coronary occlusion, complaining of chest pain. Note the high H-wave and low amplitude. The regularity and definitiveness of pattern with fairly normal stroke characteristics indicate a better mechanical myocardial function than does *A, B,* or *C.*

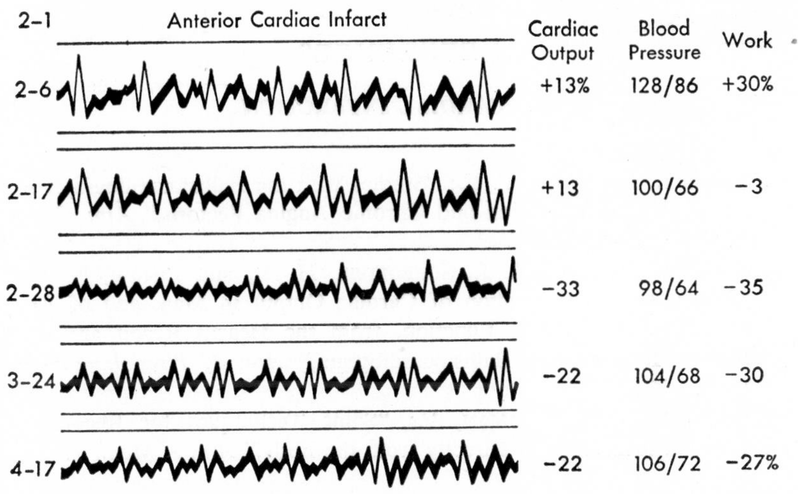


FIGURE 98. Reduction in the amplitude of the waves and, correspondingly, the relative cardiac output in a patient with an acute anterior cardiac infarct. (Starr, I., and Wood, F. C.: "Studies with Ballistocardiograph in Acute Cardiac Infarction and Chronic Angina Pectoris," *Am. Heart J.*, **25**:81, 1943.)

## REFERENCES

### MYOCARDIAL INFARCTION

1. STARR, I., and WOOD, F. C.: "Studies with the Ballistocardiograph in Acute Cardiac Infarction and Chronic Angina Pectoris," *Am. Heart J.*, **25**:81, 1943.
2. STARR, I., RAWSON, A. J., SCHROEDER, H. A., and JOSEPH, N. R.: "Studies on the Estimation of Cardiac Output in Man, and of Abnormalities in Cardiac Function, from the Heart's Recoil and the Blood's Impacts; the Ballistocardiogram," *Am. J. Physiol.*, **127**:1, 1939.
3. DOCK, W., and TAUBMAN, F.: "Some Techniques for Recording the Ballistocardiogram Directly from the Body," *Am. J. Med.*, **7**:751, 1949.

CHAPTER ELEVEN

# Angina Pectoris

THE patient's history is still of basic importance in the diagnosis of angina pectoris because of the frequent lack of objective criteria. Heberden's (*1*) original description is still classic, and when such a typical symptom complex presents itself, the diagnosis is not difficult. The history, however, is too often "atypical," and in the final analysis one can actually only question the presence of coronary artery disease.

Angina pectoris is a clinical syndrome of physiological significance, associated with many conditions and generally regarded as indicative of myocardial ischemia (*2*). It should be emphasized that while coronary arteriosclerosis is the pathological basis of angina pectoris in approximately 90 per cent of the cases, the terms are not synonymous, and that a careful search should be made for other possible mechanisms. It is also recognized that moderate coronary sclerosis can exist without signs or symptoms. Accordingly, the importance of a physiological analysis of the symptoms becomes apparent.

Numerous procedures have been proposed over the years to aid in the diagnosis of angina pectoris. They include the reproduction of pain by the injection of 1.0 cc of 1:1,000 dilution of epinephrine (*3*); a standard exercise-tolerance test in which pain is brought on by exertion (*4*); the effect of the external application of heat and cold (*5*); the demonstration of a hyperactive cardioinhibitory carotid sinus reflex (*6*); the production of the anginal syndrome by inducing general anoxemia (*7*); and the observation of electrocardiographic changes during attacks of angina pectoris as compared with those when free from pain (*8*). The above measures give evidence of the continuing search for objective aids to supplement the patient's history.

As a result of our studies we believe a new approach has been made possible by the ballistocardiograph. This instrument affords a physiological approach to a physiological problem for, as has been shown, it records mechanical heart action. The following discussion of the use of the ballistocardiograph in angina pectoris patients is presented in somewhat greater detail, since the results of the work in this particular aspect of cardiac disease appear most fruitful and commanded a considerable portion of our time.

The analysis of the records was made in the manner discussed in Chapter 4. It included consideration of the regularity, definiteness, and amplitude of the pattern, with special emphasis given to the respiratory variation. There are normally larger complexes during inspiration and smaller complexes during expiration. It is generally noted that the expiratory phase of the respiratory cycle constitutes about two thirds of the time involved. In order to express (for comparison) the degree of variation between inspiration and expiration, the respiratory variation index (RVI) is computed from the minute volume according to the following formula (*9*):

$$\text{RVI} = \frac{(\text{largest inspiratory minute volume}) \quad \text{minus} \quad (\text{smallest expiratory minute volume})}{\text{surface area}}$$

The normals were found to have an RVI between 0 and 450 cc per minute per square meter of body surface area. Any variation above 450 was considered abnormal. This is represented graphically in Figure 69.

It should be stressed that the minute volumes were calculated using Starr's original formula (*10*), which has been since modified, first by Starr and then by Tanner. This, however, does not invalidate the demonstration of an abnormal respiratory variation, since comparisons are made in the same individual, thus canceling out suc. controversial factors as the aortic diameter. Secondly, the deviation of the record from the established normal can be discussed without reference to actual cardiac output. This implies that a simplified means of demonstrating this abnormality is possible by comparing the IJ strokes to each other and to the standardization. Should Tanner's formula (*11*) be used, the limits of normalcy could be similarly established and, of course, may be different. This emphasizes the fact that our use of the RVI is an arbitrary means of demonstrating an abnormal relationship between the complexes of expiration as compared to those of inspiration—a relationship which is considered abnormal when certain arbitrary limits, determined empirically, are exceeded.

The following arbitrary grades of abnormality have been employed by us to classify the ballistocardiograms (Figure 99):

0 = normal tracing



*Grade 1*

The regularity and definitiveness are preserved. The inspiratory IJ amplitude is normal. The expiratory complexes, however, are decreased in amplitude. This accounts for the increased (abnormal) RVI.

*Grade 2*

One half or more of the complexes are abnormal, again mainly during expiration. The minute volume in this group is usually decreased owing to a decrease in the amplitude of the inspiratory complexes as well.

*Grade 3*

The complexes in both inspiration and expiration show varying degrees of abnormality in regularity and definitiveness. The complexes are still individually identifiable. The amplitude of all the complexes is low.

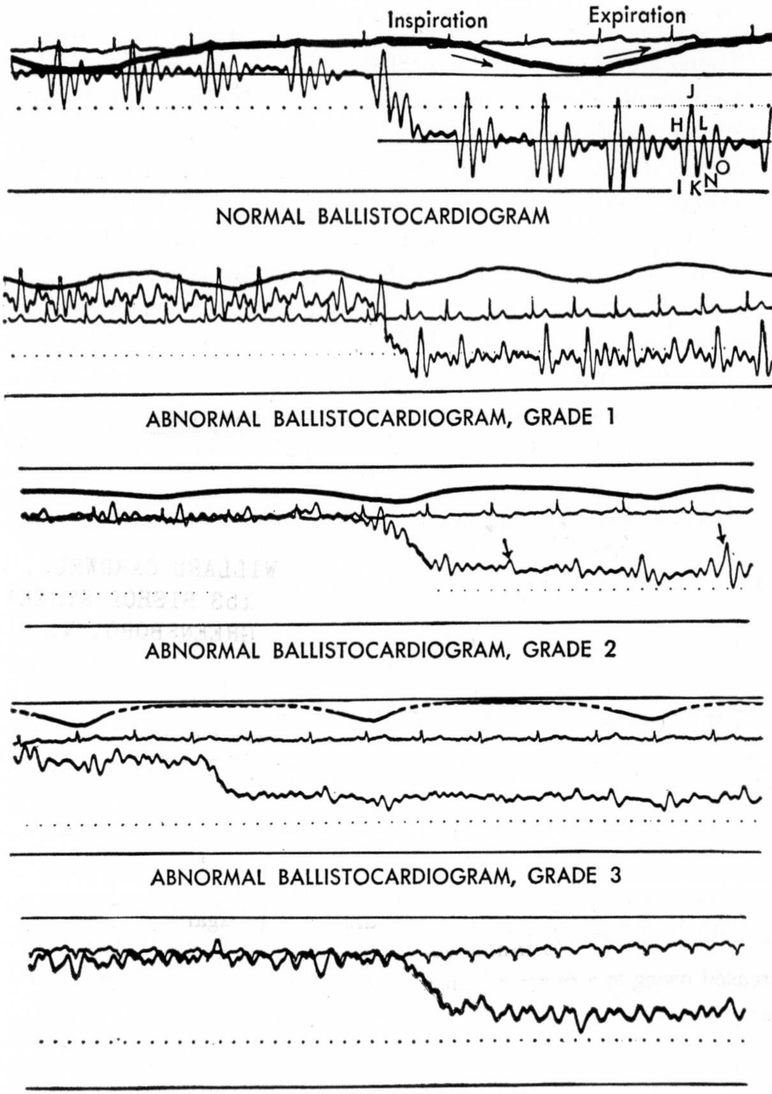


FIGURE 99. Arbitrary classification. Grades 1, increased respiratory variations with fair amplitude; 2, low amplitude and increased respiratory variation; 3, irregular expiratory complexes; 4, totally irregular and indefinite. (Brown, H. R., Jr., Hoffman, M. J., and deLalla, V., Jr.: "Ballistocardiographic Findings in Patients with Symptoms of Angina Pectoris," *Circulation,* **1**:132, 1950.)

*Grade 4*

Totally abnormal complexes are present throughout in this group. They are of low amplitude, unidentifiable, and irregular.

It should be mentioned that for the present this classification is a grouping essentially for convenience, but as patients are followed longer it may prove to be of prognostic significance. Figure 100 shows

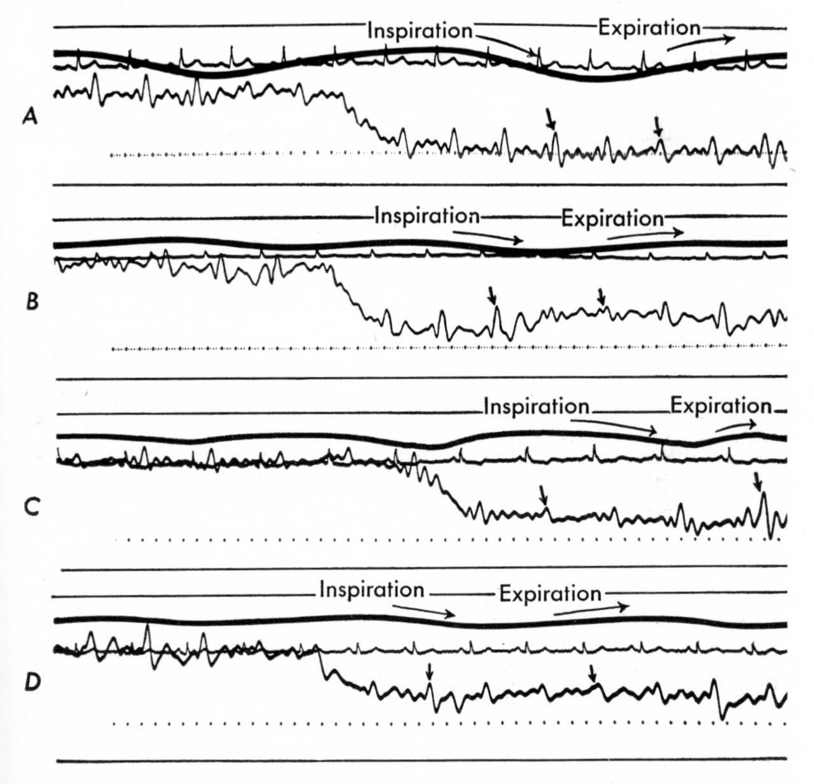


FIGURE 100. (*A*) A 51-year-old man, with normal blood pressure, who complained of precordial pain of 1 month's duration. Note the low amplitude and the increased respiratory variation (arrows), with the appearance of abnormal patterns in expiration (second arrow), characterized by shallow I- and deep K-waves. (*B*) A 58-year-old man with normal blood pressure and a 6 months' history of precordial pain on exertion. Note the marked respiratory variation (arrows), the low amplitude, and the similarity of the expiratory patterns to *A* (second

*(Caption continued on next page)*

representative patterns of patients with uncomplicated angina pectoris.

Of a total of over 250 patients with symptoms of angina, a selected series of 50 patients with uncomplicated angina has been reported (*12*). To avoid errors in analysis, patients with histories or findings of other diseases, such as hypertension, rheumatic fever, or emphysema, were excluded from this series. The findings confirmed the original observations made on a few patients with angina (*9*).

In an attempt to correlate the ballistocardiogram with the symptoms of angina pectoris, it seemed logical to divide the 50 patients into two major groups—the typical cases of angina pectoris and the atypical cases. The specific groups and their classifications were as follows:

*Group I*

Typical cases of angina pectoris
- A. Without objective evidence of cardiac abnormality.
- B. With objective evidence of cardiac abnormality.

*Group II*

Atypical cases of angina pectoris
- A. Without objective evidence of cardiac abnormality.
- B. With objective evidence of cardiac abnormality.

If a definite relationship could be established between the ballistocardiogram and those patients with angina pectoris in whom the diagnosis is beyond question, then the instrument should be of value in aiding the physician when the diagnosis is less certain.

---

arrow). (*C*) A 59-year-old woman with normal blood pressure and a 3 months' history of substernal pain. Note the low amplitude and the increased respiratory variation (arrows). Again note the appearance of abnormal waves in expiration, with shallow I- and deep K-waves (first arrow). (*D*) A 63-year-old man with normal blood pressure who has had symptoms of coronary insufficiency for 3 years and whose electrocardiograms were not remarkable. Note the very low amplitude in expiration, with the high IJ take-off and the almost absent J peak (second arrow).

The typical case embraces the following well-known symptom complex: (1) Retrosternal or precordial discomfort of a few minutes' duration. (2) The discomfort may be with or without radiation, typically to the left side of the neck, left shoulder, and down the inner aspect of the left arm, but subject to variation. (3) The pain is characteristically produced by effort, sudden exposure to cold, and emotional factors, and occasionally occurs after large meals. (4) The pain is typically relieved by rest and nitrites.

The objective evidences of cardiac abnormality include electrocardiographic changes, cardiac enlargement, heart murmurs, congestive heart failure, or a good history of such changes in the past. Patients with a history of acute coronary insufficiency have been included in Group I-B. These patients have the typical symptoms, but in addition their histories contain one or more episodes of severe cardiac pain which may be of greater duration than the typical anginal attack but without acute myocardial infarction. This type of case has recently been designated as coronary failure, a syndrome of cardiac pain intermediate between angina pectoris and acute myocardial infarction (*13*). Presumably, the underlying physiopathological mechanism of these attacks of pain is prolonged but is reversible. In this group, 5 cases of coronary thrombosis with myocardial infarction have also been included. In these cases the diagnosis was substantiated by the accepted clinical findings as well as by the typical electrocardiographic changes exhibiting acute myocardial injury and necrosis.

Group II contained the large number of cases in which the evaluation of the cardiac status was difficult because of the atypical complaints. These cases represent a diversified group; atypical because of the location of symptoms (e.g., epigastric, subscapular); atypical because of an indefinite relationship to the usual causative factors; atypical in that the predominant symptoms may be dyspnea, palpitation, fatigue, or atypical in that the discomfort may persist for more than the usual few minutes although it may be mild and not incapacitating. It is anticipated that the ballistocardiograph will lend diagnostic help in an atypical group such as this.

In this series of 50 patients 76 per cent were men at an average

age of 54 years, and 86 per cent of the members of the entire group were over 45 years of age.

The cardiac symptomatology and physical findings, the electrocardiogram, and the types of ballistocardiograms are presented in Figures 101A, 101B, 102, and 103.

The results to date have been encouraging. A relationship appears to have been established between the symptom complex of angina pectoris and the ballistocardiogram, for almost without exception the typical cases have been associated with an abnormal pattern. In the group discussed above, all 26 patients with obvious and typical angina pectoris had varying degrees of abnormality of the ballistocardiogram. Since then we have seen 1 such patient with a normal pattern. Berman, Braunstein, and McGuire (*14*) recently reported 5 normal patterns in 23 patients with angina. In the remaining 18 the ballistocardiograms were distinctly abnormal. Starr (*15*) likewise found that the ballistocardiogram "provides in the great majority of instances, either by disclosing an abnormal impact form, or by giving evidence of subnormal circulation" objective evidence to help make the diagnosis of angina pectoris. In neither of these reports was the respiratory variation taken into consideration.

Group I-A (Figure 101A) represents 5 patients in whom the diagnosis was made entirely upon the typical symptom complex. There were no objective cardiac abnormalities. The ballistocardiogram was classified as abnormal in each of these cases, illustrating the clinical usefulness of the instrument in diagnosis.

Group I-B (Figure 101B) consists of 21 cases of typical angina pectoris of varying severity with one or more positive diagnostic criteria of cardiac abnormality. At this time the question of correlation between the disease process and the degree of abnormality of the ballistocardiogram arises. It seems generally true that there is good correlation. Figure 104 shows that 5 of the patients had a history of acute myocardial infarction and 8 of acute coronary insufficiency. Of these 13 patients, 10 had a Grade 3 or 4 ballistocardiographic abnormality. This could be interpreted to mean that the symptoms of acute coronary insufficiency and acute myocardial infarction represent a more severely damaged myocardium with greater

**Group I-A: Typical Cases of Angina Pectoris without Objective Evidence of Cardiac Abnormality**

| Case Number | Patient | Age | Sex | Duration of Symptoms | *Symptoms* | | | | | Digitalis | *Physical Findings* | | | *Laboratory Findings* | |
|---|---|---|---|---|---|---|---|---|---|---|---|---|---|---|---|
| | | | | | *Acute Coronary Insufficiency* | *Myocardial Infarction* | *Angina Pectoris, Typical* | *Angina Pectoris, Atypical* | *History of Congestive Failure* | | *Blood Pressure* | *Cardiac Enlargement* | *Heart Murmurs* | *Electro-cardiogram* | *Classification of Ballisto-cardiogram* |
| | | | | *Years* | | | | | | | | | | | *Grade* |
| 1 | A. F. | 54 | F | 4½ | 0 | 0 | + | 0 | 0 | 0 | 137/70 | 0 | 0 | 0 | 1 |
| 2 | M. W. | 60 | F | 2 | 0 | 0 | + | 0 | 0 | 0 | 114/60 | 0 | 0 | 0 | 2 |
| 3 | J. F. | 55 | M | 1 | 0 | 0 | + | 0 | 0 | 0 | 130/80 | 0 | 0 | 0 | 2 |
| 4 | W. D. | 54 | M | 4½ months | 0 | 0 | + | 0 | 0 | 0 | 140/80 | 0 | 0 | 0 | 1 |
| 5 | M. O. | 51 | M | 3 months | 0 | 0 | + | 0 | 0 | 0 | 125/85 | 0 | 0 | 0 | 1 |

FIGURE 101A. (Brown, H. R., Jr., Hoffman, M. J., and deLalla, V., Jr.: "Ballistocardiographic Findings in Patients with Symptoms of Angina Pectoris," *Circulation,* **1**:132, 1950.)

**Group I-B: Typical Cases of Angina Pectoris with Objective Evidence of Cardiac Abnormality**

| Case Number | Patient | Age | Sex | Duration of Symptoms | Symptoms | | | | | Digitalis | Physical Findings | | | Laboratory Findings | |
|---|---|---|---|---|---|---|---|---|---|---|---|---|---|---|---|
| | | | | | *Acute Coronary Insufficiency* | *Myocardial Infarction* | *Angina Pectoris, Typical* | *Atypical Case* | *History of Congestive Failure* | | *Blood Pressure* | *Cardiac Enlargement* | *Heart Murmurs* | *Electro-cardiogram* | *Classification of Ballisto-cardiogram* |
| | | | | *Years* | | | | | | | | | | | *Grade* |
| 1 | J. F. | 75 | M | 3 | 0 | 0 | + | 0 | 0 | 0 | 140/80 | + | + | 0 | 3 |
| 2 | C. N. | 56 | M | 5 | 0 | 0 | + | 0 | 0 | 0 | 100/60 | 0 | 0 | + | 1 |
| 3 | A. S. | 58 | M | 2 weeks | 0 | 0 | + | 0 | 0 | 0 | 118/80 | 0 | 0 | + | 2 |
| 4 | A. P. | 64 | M | 5 months | 0 | 0 | + | 0 | 0 | 0 | 130/80 | 0 | + | + | 1 |
| 5 | O. B. | 59 | M | 6 | 0 | 0 | + | 0 | 0 | 0 | 120/72 | 0 | 0 | + | 3 |
| 6 | N. G. | 51 | M | 5 months | 0 | 0 | + | 0 | 0 | 0 | 130/90 | 0 | + | + | 2 |
| 7 | T. S. | 59 | F | 7 months | 0 | 0 | + | 0 | 0 | 0 | 100/60 | + | + | + | 2 |
| 8 | E. H. | 49 | M | 4 | 0 | 0 | + | 0 | + | + | 130/70 | + | + | + | 4 |
| 9 | F. S. | 59 | M | 10 | + | 0 | + | 0 | 0 | 0 | 100/80 | 0 | 0 | 0 | 1 |
| 10 | E. S. | 65 | M | 14 months | + | 0 | + | 0 | 0 | 0 | 160/90 | 0 | 0 | 0 | 3 |
| 11 | J. M. | 72 | F | 8 | + | 0 | + | 0 | 0 | 0 | 110/60 | + | 0 | + | 3 |
| 12 | T. C. | 70 | M | 13 | + | 0 | + | 0 | + | + | 160/80 | 0 | + | + | 2 |
| 13 | R. B. | 59 | M | 4 months | + | 0 | + | 0 | 0 | 0 | 124/88 | 0 | + | 0 | 3 |
| 14 | A. T. | 31 | M | 9 months | + | 0 | + | 0 | 0 | 0 | 120/80 | 0 | + | + | 3 |
| 15 | L. C. | 67 | F | 5 | + | 0 | + | 0 | + | + | 142/80 | + | + | + | 3 |
| 16 | J. D. | 66 | M | 2 | + | 0 | + | 0 | 0 | 0 | 130/80 | + | 0 | + | 3 |
| 17 | F. R. | 50 | M | 8 | 0 | + | + | 0 | 0 | 0 | 115/80 | 0 | 0 | + | 3 |
| 18 | L. W. | 53 | M | 6 weeks | 0 | + | + | 0 | 0 | 0 | 92/60 | 0 | 0 | + | 4 |
| 19 | L. F. | 71 | M | 3 | + | + | + | 0 | + | + | 118/80 | + | + | + | 3 |
| 20 | N. D. | 48 | M | 3 | + | + | + | 0 | + | + | 100/70 | + | + | + | 2 |
| 21 | L. C. | 53 | F | 12 weeks | 0 | + | + | 0 | + | + | 120/90 | + | + | + | 3 |

FIGURE 101B. (Brown, H. R., Jr., Hoffman, M. J., and deLalla, V., Jr.: "Ballistocardiographic Findings in Patients with Symptoms of Angina Pectoris," *Circulation,* **1**:132, 1950.)

## Group II-A: The Atypical Case without Evidence of Cardiac Abnormality

| Case Number | Patient | Age | Sex | Duration of Symptoms | Symptoms | | | | | Digitalis | Physical Findings | | | Laboratory Findings | |
|---|---|---|---|---|---|---|---|---|---|---|---|---|---|---|---|
| | | | | | *Acute Coronary Insufficiency* | *Myocardial Infarction* | *Angina Pectoris, Typical* | *Atypical Case* | *History of Congestive Failure* | | *Blood Pressure* | *Cardiac Enlargement* | *Heart Murmurs* | *Electro-cardiogram* | *Classification of Ballisto-cardiogram* |
| | | | | *Years* | | | | | | | | | | | *Grade* |
| 1 | A. S. | 53 | F | 3 | 0 | 0 | 0 | + | 0 | 0 | 140/90 | 0 | 0 | 0 | 2 |
| 2 | M. P. | 59 | M | 2 months | 0 | 0 | 0 | + | 0 | 0 | 160/80 | 0 | 0 | 0 | 3 |
| 3 | L. B. | 54 | M | 6 months | 0 | 0 | 0 | + | 0 | 0 | 116/70 | 0 | 0 | 0 | 3 |
| 4 | H. G. | 60 | M | 4 months | 0 | 0 | 0 | + | 0 | 0 | 130/84 | 0 | 0 | 0 | 1 |
| 5 | L. S. | 38 | F | 4 | 0 | 0 | 0 | + | 0 | 0 | 154/84 | 0 | 0 | 0 | 0 |
| 6 | R. B. | 25 | M | 1 | 0 | 0 | 0 | + | 0 | 0 | 150/90 | 0 | 0 | 0 | 0 |
| 7 | W. M. | 44 | M | 4 months | 0 | 0 | 0 | + | 0 | 0 | 120/80 | 0 | 0 | 0 | 1 |
| 8 | G. P. | 66 | F | 2½ | 0 | 0 | 0 | + | 0 | 0 | 125/80 | 0 | 0 | 0 | 3 |
| 9 | J. K. | 40 | M | 4 weeks | 0 | 0 | 0 | + | 0 | 0 | 120/80 | 0 | 0 | 0 | 1 |
| 10 | H. H. | 57 | M | 6 months | 0 | 0 | 0 | + | 0 | 0 | 120/80 | 0 | 0 | 0 | 2 |
| 11 | F. D. | 50 | M | 1 month | 0 | 0 | 0 | + | 0 | 0 | 132/98 | 0 | 0 | 0 | 2 |
| 12 | N. G. | 41 | M | 3 | 0 | 0 | 0 | + | 0 | 0 | 120/85 | 0 | 0 | 0 | 2 |
| 13 | H. G. | 45 | M | 1 | 0 | 0 | 0 | + | 0 | 0 | 130/90 | 0 | 0 | 0 | 0 |

FIGURE 102. (Brown, H. R., Jr., Hoffman, M. J., and deLalla, V., Jr.: "Ballistocardiographic Findings in Patients with Symptoms of Angina Pectoris," *Circulation,* **1**:132, 1950.)

## Group II-B: The Atypical Case with Evidence of Cardiac Abnormality

| Case Number | Patient | Age | Sex | Duration of Symptoms | *Symptoms* | | | | | Digitalis | *Physical Findings* | | | *Laboratory Findings* | |
|---|---|---|---|---|---|---|---|---|---|---|---|---|---|---|---|
| | | | | | *Acute Coronary Insufficiency* | *Myocardial Infarction* | *Angina Pectoris, Typical* | *Atypical Case* | *History of Congestive Failure* | | *Blood Pressure* | *Cardiac Enlargement* | *Heart Murmurs* | *Electro-cardiogram* | *Classification of Ballisto-cardiogram* |
| | | | | *Years* | | | | | | | | | | | *Grade* |
| 1 | W. Z. | 60 | M | 1 | 0 | 0 | 0 | + | 0 | 0 | 125/85 | + | 0 | 0 | 1 |
| 2 | M. L. | 51 | F | 1 | 0 | 0 | 0 | + | 0 | + | 130/85 | + | 0 | 0 | 2 |
| 3 | C. S. | 46 | M | 1½ | 0 | 0 | 0 | + | 0 | 0 | 130/90 | 0 | + | 0 | 2 |
| 4 | H. E. | 29 | M | 2 | 0 | 0 | 0 | + | 0 | 0 | 120/70 | 0 | + | 0 | 1 |
| 5 | M. P. | 52 | F | 2½ | 0 | 0 | 0 | + | 0 | 0 | 130/80 | 0 | 0 | + | 4 |
| 6 | A. S. | 42 | F | 2 | + | 0 | 0 | + | + | + | 110/70 | 0 | 0 | + | 3 |
| 7 | E. S. | 55 | M | 4 | 0 | 0 | 0 | + | 0 | 0 | 100/50 | 0 | 0 | + | 2 |
| 8 | E. P. | 56 | M | 5 months | 0 | 0 | 0 | + | 0 | 0 | 140/90 | 0 | 0 | + | 1 |
| 9 | J. L. | 47 | M | 3 months | 0 | 0 | 0 | + | 0 | 0 | 150/85 | + | 0 | + | 2 |
| 10 | W. B. | 66 | M | 2 | 0 | 0 | 0 | + | 0 | 0 | 154/64 | + | + | + | 3 |
| 11 | C. M. | 87 | M | 2 | 0 | 0 | 0 | + | 0 | 0 | 120/80 | + | + | + | 1 |

FIGURE 103. (Brown, H. R., Jr., Hoffman, M. J., and deLalla, V., Jr.: "Ballistocardiographic Findings in Patients with Symptoms of Angina Pectoris," *Circulation,* **1**:132, 1950.)

**Statistical Summary**

| | *Typical Cases of Angina Pectoris* | | | | *Atypical Cases* | |
|---|---|---|---|---|---|---|
| | | *I-B—with Cardiac Abnormality* | | | | |
| | *I-A—without Cardiac Abnormality* | *Entire Group* | *With Acute Coronary Insufficiency* | *With Acute Myocardial Infarction* | *II-A—without Cardiac Abnormality* | *II-B—with Cardiac Abnormality* |
| Number of cases | 5 | 21 | 8 | 5 | 13 | 11 |
| Men | 3 | 17 | 6 | 4 | 10 | 8 |
| Women | 2 | 4 | 2 | 1 | 3 | 3 |
| Cardiac enlargement | 0 | 9 | 3 | 3 | 0 | 5 |
| Heart murmurs | 0 | 12 | 4 | 3 | 0 | 4 |
| Positive electrocardiogram | 0 | 17 | 5 | 5 | 0 | 7 |
| Positive ballistocardiogram | 5 | 21 | 8 | 5 | 10 | 11 |
| Grade 1 | 3 | 3 | 1 | 0 | 3 | 4 |
| Grade 2 | 2 | 5 | 1 | 1 | 4 | 4 |
| Grade 3 | 0 | 11 | 6 | 3 | 3 | 2 |
| Grade 4 | 0 | 2 | 0 | 1 | 0 | 1 |

FIGURE 104. (Brown, H. R., Jr., Hoffman, M. J., and deLalla, V., Jr.: "Ballistocardiographic Findings in Patients with Symptoms of Angina Pectoris," *Circulation,* **1**:132, 1950.)

impairment in contractile power (*16*). Only 3 of 13 patients without acute episodes had ballistocardiograms classified above Grade 2, although all were abnormal.

An atypical group of cases where the diagnosis was suspected was studied in a similar manner. Groups II-A and II-B (Figures 102 and 103) include 24 such cases. Of these groups, 21 patients showed varying degrees of abnormality of the ballistocardiogram, although only 11 of the 21 had one or more of the usual stigmata of cardiovascular abnormality. Three patients with no other objective evidence of cardiac abnormality and with normal ballistocardiograms were thought at the time to be suffering from anxiety states. Subsequent evaluation of these cases seems to substantiate this conclusion. It should be remembered that the patients in this group were those clinically suspected of having heart disease but in whom sufficient corroborative evidence was lacking. In view of the previous evidence the ballistocardiographic abnormalities in these two groups give support to the diagnosis of angina pectoris.

It appears that there is a definite relationship between the typical symptom complex of angina pectoris and an abnormal ballistocardiogram, which allows the ballistocardiograph to be used as a diagnostic aid in atypical cases of angina pectoris.

Berman, Braunstein, and McGuire (*14*) described another possible diagnostic test for angina pectoris which utilizes the ballistocardiograph. In normal individuals there is a significant increase in cardiac output following meals. In their series the cardiac output was calculated from the ballistocardiograms. The controls showed a 1.4-liter (24 per cent) increase in cardiac output 30 min following meals. The patients with angina pectoris, whose pattern was sufficiently normal so that cardiac output could be calculated, failed to show any significant change (Figure 105). Figure 106, *A* and *B,* illustrates their typical ballistocardiographic findings before and 30 min following a meal in a normal individual and in a patient with severe angina. These investigators suggest that this inability of patients with angina pectoris to increase their cardiac output after a meal might be utilized further to evaluate the cardiac state in such patients.

It is of interest to note in the 50 cases just discussed that the duration of symptoms in the atypical cases was 17.3 months as compared

**Ballistocardiographic Changes Before and Following Meals in Patients with Angina, Not in Congestive Failure, and in Control Subjects**

| *Before Meals (Liters per Minute) Angina (Not in Congestive Failure)* | *30 Minutes Following Meals (Liters per Minute)* |
|---|---|
| 8.4 | 8.2 |
| 5.7 | 5.1 |
| 5.2 | 4.8 |
| 6.9 | 7.0 |
| 6.7 | 6.5 |
| 32.9 | 31.6 (—4 per cent) |
| Controls | |
| 5.8 | 6.6 |
| 4.1 | 7.7 |
| 7.1 | 6.5 |
| 5.8 | 6.1 |
| 6.0 | 8.4 |
| 4.8 | 6.6 |
| 34.6 | 42.9 (+24 per cent) |

FIGURE 105. Note that the normal cardiac output increased following a meal, whereas it decreased in the angina patients. (Berman, B., Braunstein, J. R., and McQuire, J.: "The Effects of Meals on the Electrocardiogram and Ballistocardiogram in Patients with Angina Pectoris," *Circulation,* **1**:1017, 1950.)

to 39.2 months for the typical cases (excluding the 5 patients with acute myocardial infarctions). This suggests that many patients with coronary artery disease may have atypical complaints preceding the development of classic and easily recognizable symptoms.

It is also an accepted belief that a considerable number of patients may present no signs or symptoms, yet there may be a moderate degree of arteriosclerosis (*17*). The patient who ultimately suffers an acute myocardial infarction "who never had a sick day in his life" may be in this category. It is suggested that this group, devoid of symptoms or known stigmata of cardiovascular abnormality but discovered to have abnormal ballistocardiograms, may be regarded as predisposed to angina pectoris or coronary thrombosis. The implications of the ability to detect those predisposed is obvious. Impetus for such a study can be found in the 8- to 10-year after-histories secured by Starr (*18*) on 90 supposedly healthy individuals over 40

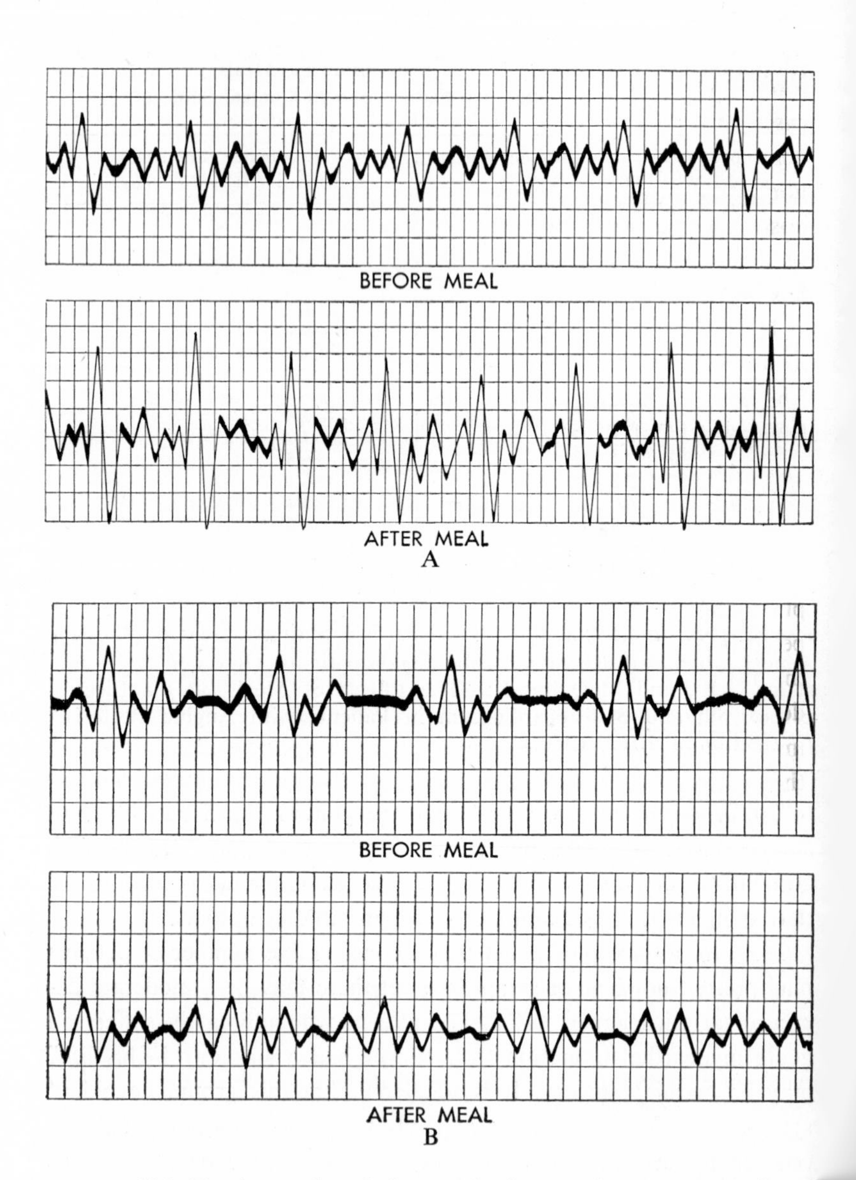


FIGURE 106. Tracings taken before and after meals on a normal and an angina patient. (*A*) Normal subject. Ballistocardiograms, made before and 30 minutes following a meal, showing normal response to meal with increase in cardiac output. The patient, C.G., was a nurse 52

years of age previously tested for the purpose of compiling normal standards. Of these subjects, 4 had ballistocardiograms abnormal in form, and 3 of the 4 developed coronary heart disease. Six other cases with abnormally small complexes also subsequently developed coronary artery disease. Starr concludes: "A ballistocardiogram abnormal in form, or of unusually small amplitude, is of serious prognostic significance. The ballistocardiographic method gives promise of identifying coronary heart disease far earlier in its course than has been possible hitherto."

It must be emphasized that "angina pectoris" is a symptom, and its absence does not exclude the diagnosis of coronary artery disease. The common finding of abnormal ballistocardiograms in supposedly healthy individuals over 50 years of age is not surprising when the incidence of heart disease is recalled (*19*). It would seem from the empirical data presented that the ballistocardiogram will furnish objective evidence of circulatory abnormality in such cases.

The possible relationship of abnormal blood pooling (diminished pulmonary pool, secondary to increased splanchnic pool) to angina pectoris has been reported (*20*). This concept is well illustrated by the history of Mrs. P., a hypertensive woman who underwent bilateral dorsal sympathectomy. She developed precordial chest pain almost immediately after the operation; upon questioning, she stated that the pain was brought on by passive standing, relieved slightly by mild exertion, but relieved maximally by lying down with the legs elevated. Her ballistocardiogram showed a marked diminution of amplitude and an increased respiratory variation postoperatively. It was believed that the great amount of splanchnic and leg pooling that occurred on standing had diminished the pulmonary pool and left ventricular output at critical levels, accounting for the increased res-

---

years of age. She had no organic heart disease. (*B*) Patient with angina. Ballistocardiograms, made before and 30 minutes following a meal, showing decrease in cardiac output. The patient was a 53-year-old white machinist with severe angina. He died while asleep. (Berman, B., Braunstein, J. R., and McGuire, J.: "The Effects of Meals on the Electrocardiogram and Ballistocardiogram in Patients with Angina Pectoris." *Circulation,* **1**:1017, 1950.)

piratory variation and the angina. This led to the use of abdominal and leg binders in an attempt to decrease the amount of pooling. When these binders were worn she experienced relief of her chest pain, and her ballistocardiogram improved, with a return of the respiratory variation toward normal (i.e., diminution of variation). This same phenomena also occurred in other patients; Figure 107 shows the traces obtained in one such patient.

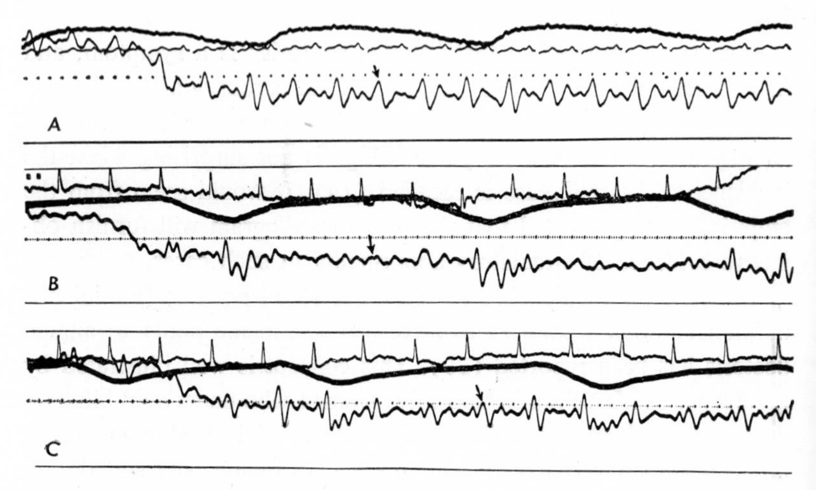


Sympathectomy—Reversal of Respiratory Variation with Binders

FIGURE 107. Three records taken on a hypertensive patient before (*A*) and 2 weeks after (*B* and *C*) a dorsal sympathectomy. Tracing *B* was taken without abdominal binders or elastic stockings. Note the marked decrease of amplitude of the expiratory patterns (arrow) as compared with *A*, and the consequent increase of respiratory variation. Tracing *C* was taken immediately after tracing *B*, but with a rigid abdominal support and elastic stockings applied. Note the increase in the amplitude of the expiratory beats (arrow) as compared with *B*. The sensitivity of the ballistocardiograph amplifier was kept constant for tracings *B* and *C*. (Brown, H. R., Jr., and deLalla, V., Jr.: "The Ballistocardiogram, Description and Clinical Use," *Am. J. Med.*, **9**:718, 1950.)

Although the concept of abnormal splanchnic and leg pooling as a possible cause of angina was independently arrived at in this laboratory (*20*), a subsequent review of the literature revealed numerous articles stating essentially the same thing. Kerr has reported on cases of angina pectoris which he felt were due to abnormal posture and abdominal ptosis (*21* through *26*). These obese patients were helped by an abdominal belt. It was also Kerr's opinion that the symptoms of angina were secondary to decreased venous return with reduced filling of the coronaries. He treated over 300 cases with belts and reported uniformly good results. This improvement with belt therapy in patients with angina pectoris has been reported by others (*27* and *28*).

The ballistocardiogram lends itself well to the evaluation and selection of those angina patients who might be expected to improve with belt therapy. This can be done in the following manner: records are taken on the same patient before and after the application of an abdominal belt; any change in amplitude is noted, and the respiratory variation index is calculated. If there is an improvement with the belt, then the patient may be considered a candidate for belt therapy (Figure 108). Thus far, over 160 patients have been screened

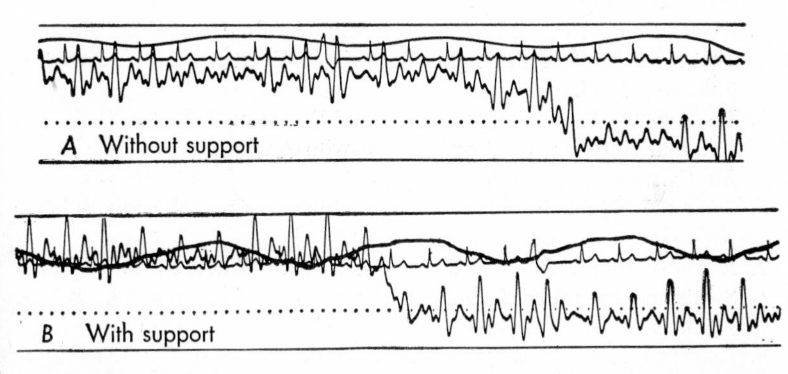


FIGURE 108. Tracings taken on a patient with angina pectoris. *A* shows increased respiratory variation without the belt. *B* shows the effect of abdominal support. Note the reduced respiratory variation.

in this fashion, and approximately 30 per cent (51 patients) have shown an improved ballistocardiogram with the belt. Of these 51 patients, 31 accepted the recommendation, and wore the belt as prescribed, and 18 of these returned for adequate follow-up studies; 13 of the 18 patients on whom follow-up studies were obtained showed definite clinical and ballistocardiographic improvement with the belt, and 5 showed no improvement. The duration of treatment varies from 2 to 24 months. It is admitted that the series is small and of too short a duration to make definite conclusions possible, yet the results are encouraging and warrant continuation of the procedure.

## REFERENCES

### ANGINA PECTORIS


1. HEBERDEN, W.: "Some Account of a Disorder of the Breast," *Med. Tr. Roy. Coll. Physicians,* **2**:58, 1772.
2. KEEFER, C. S., and RESNICK, W. H.: "Angina Pectoris: A Syndrome Caused by Anoxemia of the Myocardium," *Arch. Int. Med.,* **41**:769, 1928.
3. LEVINE, S. A., ERNSTENE, A. C., and JACOBSON, B. M.: "The Use of Epinephrine as a Diagnostic Test for Angina Pectoris," *Arch. Int. Med.,* **45**:191, 1930.
4. RISEMAN, J. E. F., and STERN, B.: "Standardized Exercise Tolerance Test for Patients with Angina Pectoris on Exertion," *Am. J. M. Sc.,* **188**:646, 1934.
5. FREEDBERG, A. A., SPIEGL, E. D., and RISEMAN, J. E. F.: "Effect of External Heat and Cold on Patients with Angina Pectoris: Evidence for Existence of a Reflex Factor," *Am. Heart J.,* **27**:611, 1944.
6. SIGLER, L. H.: "Hyperactive Cardioinhibitory Carotid Sinus Reflex," *Arch. Int. Med.,* **67**:177, 1941.
7. ROTHCHILD, M. A., and KISSEN, M.: "Production of the Anginal Syndrome by Induced General Anoxemia," *Am. Heart J.,* **8**:729, 1933.
8. RISEMAN, J. E. F., WALLER, J. W., and BROWN, M. G.: "The Electrocardiogram during Attacks of Angina Pectoris; Characteristics and Diagnostic Significance," *Am. Heart J.,* **19**:683, 1940.
9. BROWN, H. R., JR., and DELALLA, V., JR.: "The Ballistocardiogram, Description and Clinical Use," *Am. J. Med.,* **9**:718, 1950.
10. STARR, I., RAWSON, A. J., SCHROEDER, H. A., and JOSEPH, N. R.: "Studies on the Estimation of Cardiac Output in Man, and of Abnormalities in Cardiac Function, from the Heart's Recoil and the Blood's Impacts; the Ballistocardiogram," *Am. J. Physiol.,* **127**:1, 1939.
11. TANNER, J. M.: "The Construction of Normal Standards for Cardiac Output in Man," *J. Clin. Investigation,* **28**:567, 1949.

12. BROWN, H. R., JR., HOFFMAN, M. J., and DELALLA, V., JR.: "Ballistocardiographic Findings in Patients with Symptoms of Angina Pectoris," *Circulation,* **1**:132, 1950.
13. FREEDBERG, A. A., BLUMGART, H. L., ZOLL, P. M., and SCHLESINGER, M. J.: "Coronary Failure. The Syndrome of Cardiac Pain Intermittent between Angina Pectoris and Acute Myocardial Infarction," *J.A.M.A.,* **138**:107, 1948.
14. BERMAN, B., BRAUNSTEIN, J. R., and MCGUIRE, J.: "The Effects of Meals on the Electrocardiogram and the Ballistocardiogram in Patients with Angina Pectoris," *Circulation,* **1**:1017, 1950.
15. STARR, I., and WOOD, F. C.: "Studies with the Ballistocardiograph in Acute Cardiac Infarction and Chronic Angina Pectoris," *Am. Heart J.,* **25**:81, 1943.
16. TENNANT, R., and WIGGERS, C. J.: "The Effect of Coronary Occlusion on the Myocardial Contraction," *Am. J. Physiol.,* **112**:351, 1935.
17. *Nomenclature and Criteria for Diagnosis of Diseases of the Heart,* 4th ed., J. J. Little and Ives Company, New York, 1943, p. 36.
18. STARR, I.: "On the Later Development of Heart Disease in Apparently Healthy Persons with Abnormal Ballistocardiograms. Eight to Ten Years After-Histories of 90 Persons over 40 Years of Age," *Am. J. M. Sc.,* **214**:233, 1947.
19. BROWN, H. R., JR., and PEARSON, R.: "Seasonal Variations in Heart and Coronary Disease as Related to Various Environmental Factors," *Am. Heart J.,* **35**:763, 1948.
20. DELALLA, V., JR., and BROWN, H. R., JR.: "The Respiratory Variation of the Ballistocardiogram," *Am. J. Med.,* **9**:728, 1950.
21. KERR, W. J., and LAGEN, J. B.: "The Postural Syndrome Related to Obesity Leading to Postural Emphysema and Cardio-Respiratory Failure," *Ann. Int. Med.,* **10**:569, 1936.
22. KERR, W. J., and LAGEN, J. B.: "A Supporting Elastic Belt for Use in Abdominal Obesity (Postural Syndrome)," *J. Lab. Clin. Med.,* **22**:1121, 1937.
23. KERR, W. J.: "The Treatment of Angina Pectoris by Methods Which Appear to Promote More Adequate Filling of the Heart," *Am. Heart J.,* **16**:544, 1938.
24. KERR, W. J., CANNON, E. F., and LAGEN, J. B.: "A New Approach to the Etiology and Treatment of Angina Pectoris," *Tr. A. Am. Physicians,* **54**:225, 1939.
25. KERR, W. J.: "Angina Pectoris, Etiology and Treatment," *Texas State J. Med.,* **37**:711, 1942.
26. KERR, W. J.: "Faulty Movements of the Diaphragm as a Cause of

Non-Obstructive Emphysema and Angina Pectoris," *Radiology,* **39**:153, 1942.

27. LEVINE, S. A.: *Clinical Heart Disease,* 3rd ed., W. B. Saunders Company, Philadelphia, 1945, 462 pp.
28. KERR, W. J., CANNON, E. F., and LAGEN, J. B.: "A New Approach to the Etiology and Treatment of Angina Pectoris," *Tr. A. Am. Physicians,* **54**:225, 1939. (See comments by Dr. H. L. Alexander.)

## CHAPTER TWELVE

# Congestive Failure

THE ballistocardiogram usually is abnormal in cases of congestive failure, with irregular, indefinite patterns of low amplitude. The main exceptions to this are found in high-output failure, such as may occur with anemia or hyperthyroidism. Figure 109 shows an example of

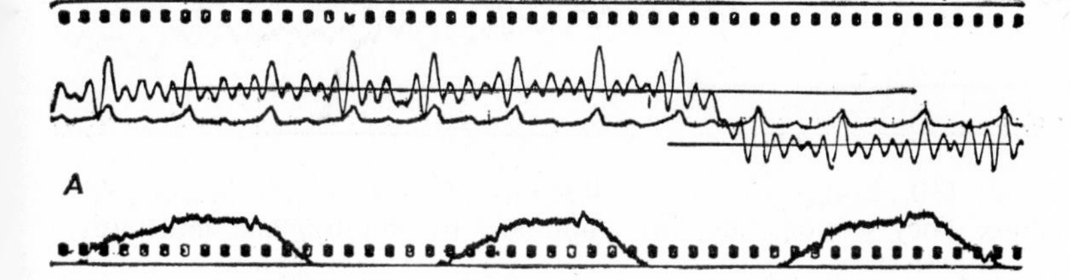


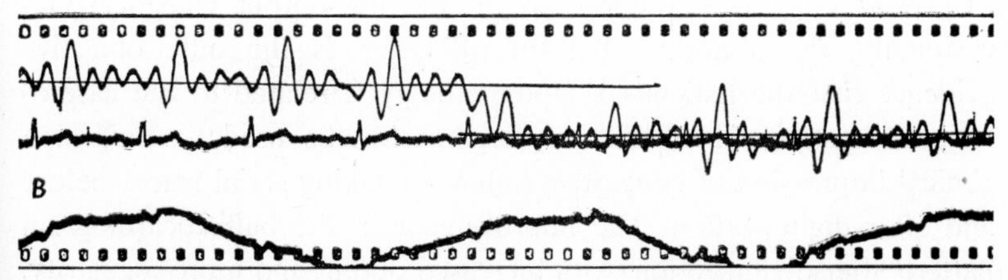


FIGURE 109. Records of an adult male who had leg edema, without dyspnea or heart murmurs. Tracing *A* was taken before digitalization. It has fairly normal characteristics and is of good amplitude. The minute volume was calculated to be 4,325 cc. *B* was taken after digitalization. Note the increased amplitude of pattern. The minute volume was calculated to be 4,960 cc.

mild congestive failure in a man whose pattern was of good amplitude and of fairly normal characteristics. His leg edema disappeared, and his calculated output improved slightly following digitalization (see legend, Figure 109).

However, the most frequent finding in congestive failure is a pattern of low amplitude, with minimal to marked irregularity which improves upon treatment (Figure 110). This may be related to the concept

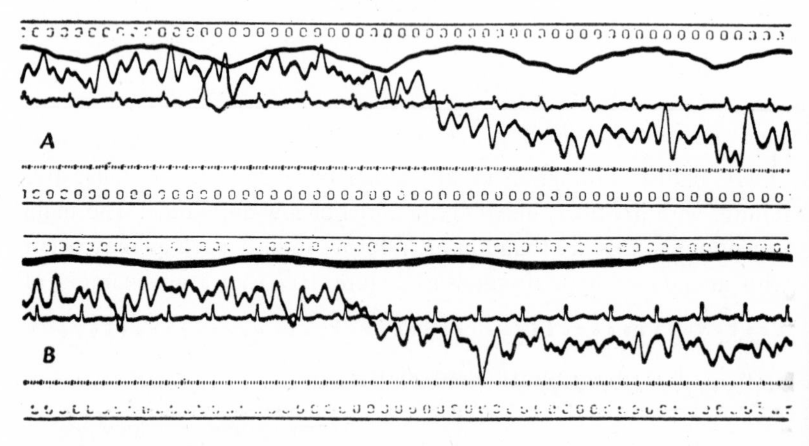


FIGURE 110. Congestive failure. Records of two patients in congestive failure. They demonstrate low amplitude, irregularity, and indefinitiveness of pattern.

that most congestive failures are in the low-output category. Occasionally, the abnormal ballistocardiogram is the only objective evidence that the patient's symptomatology is related to the cardiovascular system. The ballistocardiogram can be used to confirm a clinical impression of congestive failure by taking serial traces before and after digitalization. The improvement of the ballistocardiogram pattern after digitalization, with increased output and more regularity, is good evidence that the patient had been in cardiac failure (Figure 111, *A* and *B*). Three case histories which demonstrate these points follow.

1. Mrs. P. was a 62-year-old neurotic woman who complained of dyspnea on exertion. Neither the electrocardiogram nor physical

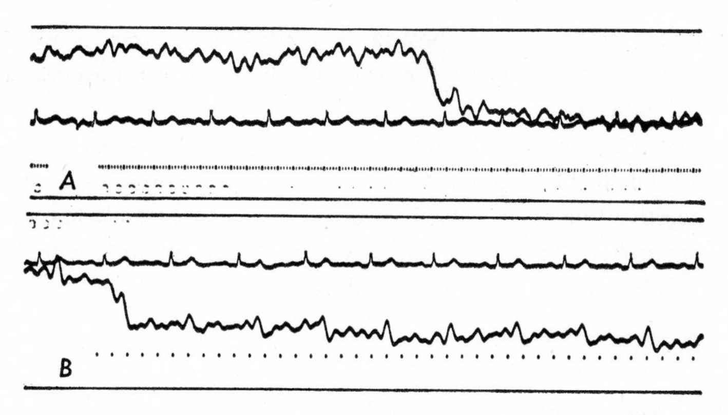


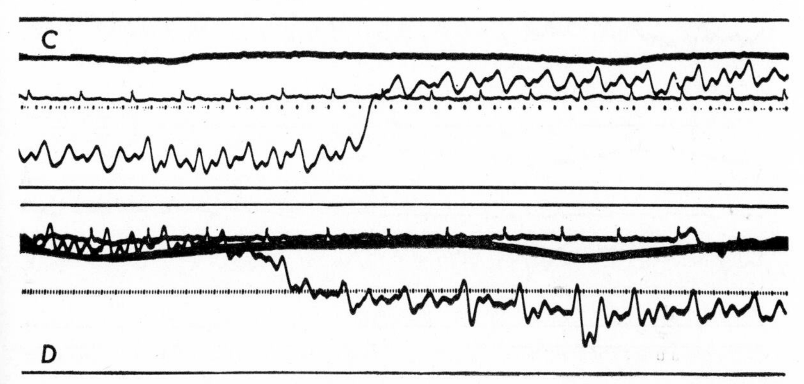


FIGURE 111. *A* and *B* are serial records on a 48-year-old woman who had congestive failure. Tracing *A* shows the typical irregular, indefinite pattern of low amplitude. Tracing *B* was taken after digitalization. Note the improved output and the return of definitiveness and regularity. *C* and *D* were taken on a 62-year-old neurotic woman who complained of dyspnea. The electrocardiograms were not helpful, nor were the physical signs. Tracing *C* showed that the heart was definitely pathological; the output was very low, and there were indications of minimal irregularity of pattern. This strongly suggested an early failure, and digitalization was instituted. Tracing *D* was taken after digitalization. Note the improved output and the return of regularity and definitiveness. The pattern characteristics remain abnormal. (Trace *B* from Brown, H. R., Jr., and deLalla, V., Jr.: "The Ballistocardiogram, Description and Clinical Use," *Am. J. Med.*, **9**:718, 1950.)

findings were helpful. The ballistocardiogram revealed an abnormal pattern of low amplitude, with minimal indications of irregularity suggesting early cardiac failure (Figure 111, *C*). For this reason she was digitalized, and she improved. Tracing 111, *D*, was taken after digitalization and showed an improved output and a return of regularity of pattern.

2. Mr. E. is a 51-year-old male who had been complaining of slight dyspnea on exertion; there were no other objective physical signs of congestive failure. A ballistocardiogram was taken and showed an irregular pattern of low amplitude which was compatible with congestive failure (Figure 112, *A*). He was digitalized; note the improvement of symptoms and ballistocardiogram pattern (Figure 112, *B*).

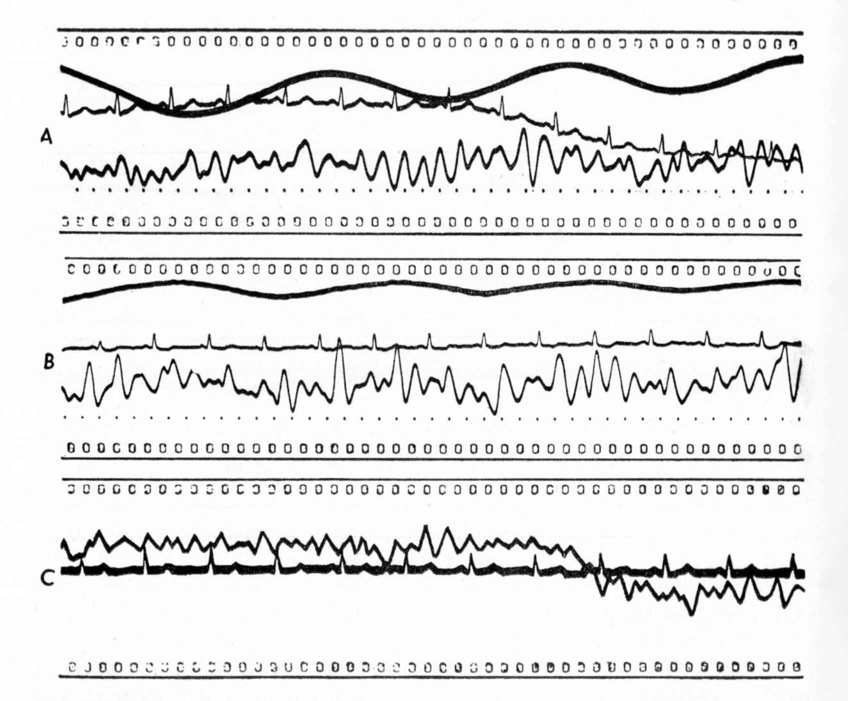


FIGURE 112. Congestive failure. *A* and *B* are on the same patient. *A* is predigitalis. Note the improved pattern in *B* following digitalis. *C* is a record of a male who had only leg edema. Note the low amplitude and irregular pattern.

3. Mr. C. is a 59-year-old male who developed leg edema without any evidence of cardiac abnormality or any history of dyspnea. A ballistocardiogram revealed markedly abnormal heart action and led to his digitalization (Figure 112, *C*).

CHAPTER THIRTEEN



# Rheumatic Heart Disease

In some respects the ballistocardiogram findings in rheumatic heart disease have not been so striking as those in other types of heart disease. The only findings reported by others are those of Starr, who stated that 8 per cent of 100 patients with subnormal circulation were rheumatics (*1* and *2*). No truly specific changes, such as the K-wave deepening seen in hypertension, have been demonstrated with certainty. Our experience with the ballistocardiogram in acute and chronic rheumatic heart disease is based on studies of 94 patients; of these, 13 had a previous attack of acute rheumatic fever without subsequent clinical heart disease; 8 had possible, and 7 had definite acute rheumatic fever; 8 had possible rheumatic heart disease, and the rest had definite chronic rheumatic heart disease.

## Acute Rheumatic Fever

Most patients with definite acute rheumatic myocarditis will show some abnormalities in their ballistocardiograms, although the changes may not be great (Figure 113). The H-K time is usually inconstant, the record is a little irregular, and the L-waves are shallow.

We have taken records on 8 patients with suspected and 7 patients with definite acute rheumatic fever. Of the former 8 patients, 4 had normal ballistocardiograms, and of the latter group only 1 had an entirely normal record. The degree of ballistocardiogram abnormality in acute rheumatic fever varies with the severity of the attack. The

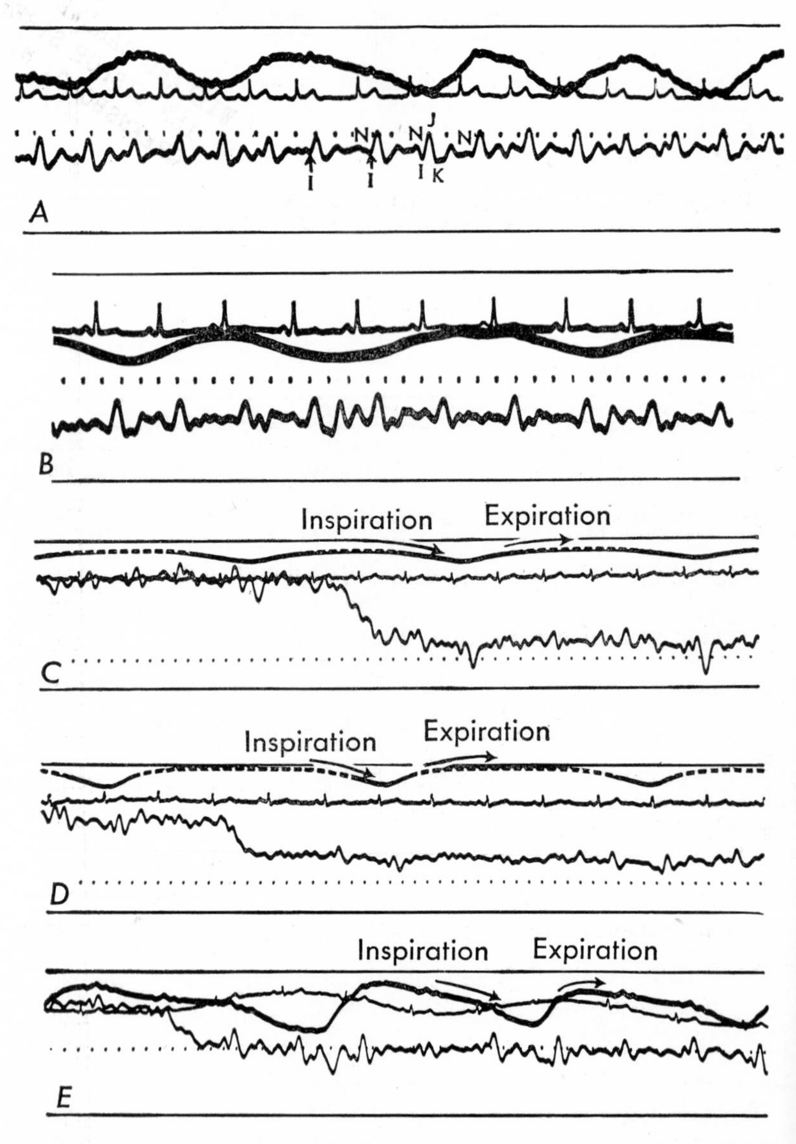


FIGURE 113. *A* and *B* are records of two young patients with acute rheumatic fever. Note the slight irregularity of pattern. *C, D,* and *E* are serial tracings on a 45-year-old man who had purpura, fever, malaise, and tachycardia. Note the low amplitude and irregular and indefinite complexes of tracing *C*. The electrocardiogram was not remarkable.

**Ballistocardiogram Patterns in Seven Cases of Acute Rheumatic Fever**

6 Showed abnormal pattern characteristics
4 Were irregular
3 Were indefinite
3 Showed moderate increased respiratory variation
3 Showed inconstant H-K times
1 Was of low amplitude

FIGURE 114

observations we have made in 7 cases of definite acute rheumatic fever are summarized in Figure 114. Only 1 of the 7 patients had a perfectly normal tracing. The commonest abnormality was a change in the pattern configuration of the beats, since 6 of the 7 showed this. The most frequent change was shallowness of the I-waves (Figure 113, *A*), but some also showed deep K-waves. Approximately half of the group had slight irregularity or loss of definitiveness of the complexes (Figure 113, *B*). Probably extensive myocardial involv-ment must be present before the cardiac function will change enough to produce a very irregular ballistocardiogram, such as is seen in Figure 113, *C*. Half of the group showed a variable H-K time. This interval is normally constant to within 0.02 sec, regardless of the heart rate. A variable H-K time will be seen in any condition which greatly disturbs myocardial function.

There were 8 patients with suspected acute rheumatic carditis; 4 of these had normal ballistocardiograms, 1 had a somewhat irregular pattern, 2 showed some increase in respiratory variation (1 of these had occasional deep K-waves, and the other some shallow K's), and 1 showed only slightly deepened K-waves. All of these patients had constant H-K times.

---

The very abnormal ballistocardiogram aided in making a diagnosis of acute rheumatic myocarditis. As the patient improved, the ballistocardio-gram improved, until on the day of discharge (tracing *E*) the output was nearly normal and the pattern had become regular and definite; the pattern characteristics remained abnormal.

**Chronic Rheumatic Heart Disease**

We have taken records on 79 patients with inactive rheumatic heart disease. Of these, the diagnosis of rheumatic heart disease was questionable in 8 patients, all of whom had borderline tracings; 12 had a history of rheumatic fever, but no evidence of heart disease, and 10 of these had normal records; the other 2 had abnormal records. Of those with definite rheumatic heart disease, 15 patients had normal ballistocardiograms, 31 had slightly abnormal records, 15 had moderately abnormal records, and 12 showed marked abnormalities in their tracings.

The ballistocardiogram pattern may be nearly normal in chronic rheumatic heart disease (Figures 115 and 116) or may be markedly

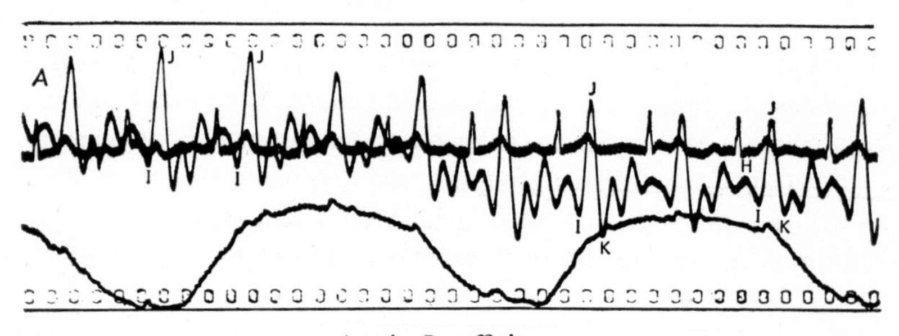


Aortic Insufficiency

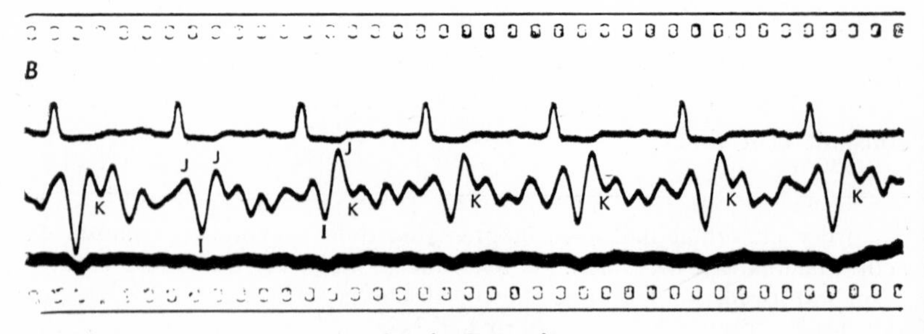


Aortic Stenosis

FIGURE 115. Rheumatic heart disease. Note the large amplitude in aortic insufficiency, and the deep I- and shallow K-waves of aortic stenosis.

abnormal, depending upon the amount of myocardial damage and the presence of complicating factors such as auricular fibrillation (Figure 116, *C*), or congestive failure (Figures 117 and 118).

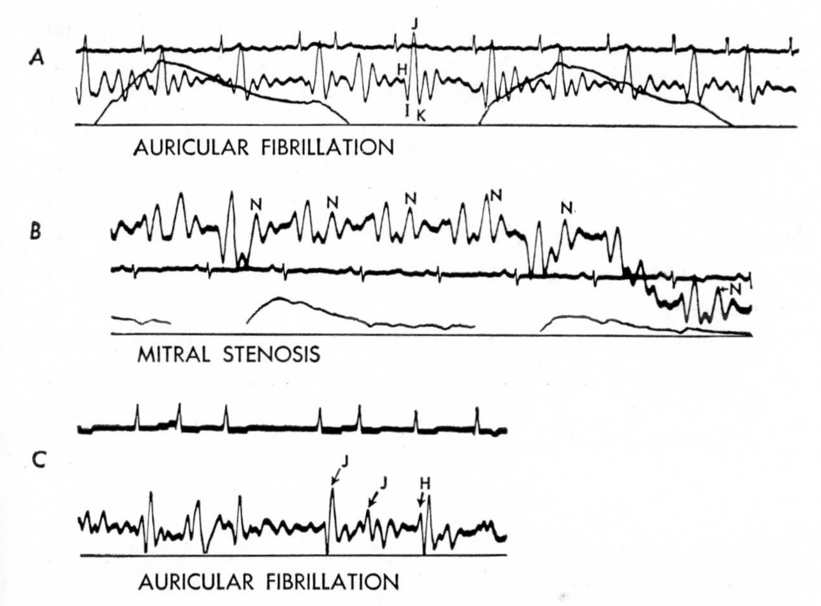


FIGURE 116. Three records of patients with rheumatic heart disease. *A* shows a pattern of auricular fibrillation where the ballistocardiogram amplitude and characteristics are within normal limits; note the small H-waves. *B* shows high N peaks in a case with mitral stenosis. *C* is a pattern of a patient with auricular fibrillation. Note the abnormal patterns of low amplitude occurring with beats where the filling time was short (compare first labeled J peak with second J peak).

There are no well-established specific changes in chronic rheumatic valvulitis. In aortic insufficiency the amplitude is usually greatly increased (Figure 115, *A*), owing possibly to the compensatory large stroke volume or to increased pulse pressure or both. In aortic stenosis we have observed shallow K-waves such as are seen in coarctation (Figure 115, *B*). This is to be expected since the stenotic valve interferes with proper transmission of the pulse wave.

We have seen high N-waves in 3 of 10 cases of mitral stenosis (Figure 116, *B*) and high L-waves in 3 of these patients. In 5 patients

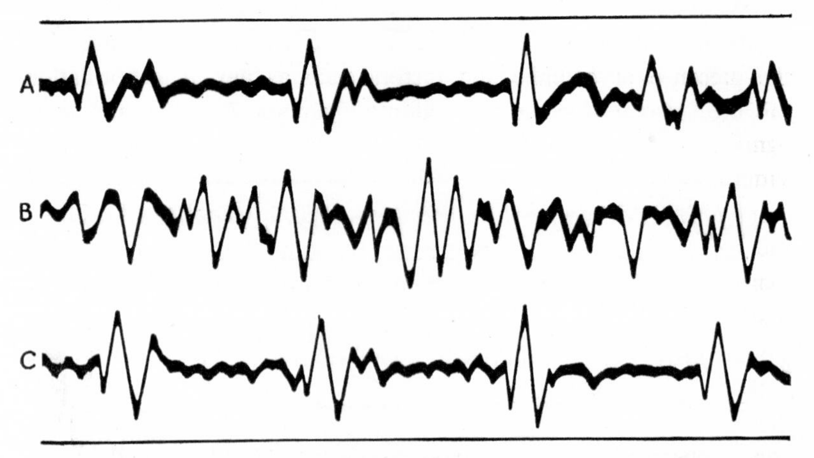

Digitalis Effect

FIGURE 117. Records showing the effects of withdrawal of digitalis in a patient with rheumatic heart disease who was fibrillating. *A* shows the record when the patient was fully digitalized. *B* shows the record 14 days after digitalis was stopped; at this time there were no clinical signs of congestive failure; note the reduced amplitude and the increased irregularity of pattern. *C* shows the pattern after 2.0 gm of digitalis had been given. (Starr, I.: "Clinical Studies with the Ballistocardiograph," *Am. J. M. Sc.*, **202**:469, 1941.)

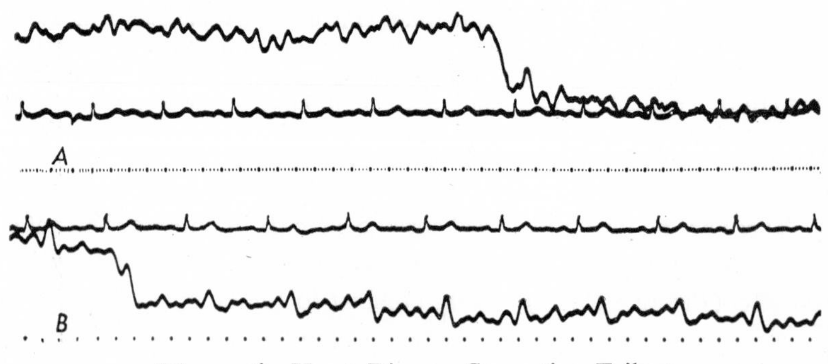

Rheumatic Heart Disease Congestive Failure

FIGURE 118. Two records of a patient with rheumatic heart disease in congestive failure (*A*) and out of congestive failure (*B*). Note the improved amplitude and regularity of pattern following digitalization. (Brown, H. R., Jr., and deLalla, V., Jr.: "The Ballistocardiogram, Description and Clinical Use," *Am. J. Med.*, **9**:718, 1950.)

with mitral stenosis and an aortic lesion, 2 had high N-waves, and 1 had high L-waves. These observations are quite suggestive, but their significance is as yet unknown. Auricular fibrillation may cause the pattern to be abnormal, especially if the ventricular rate is rapid (Figure 116, *C*). H-waves will be small or absent (Figure 116, *A* and *C*). This is not surprising since auricular systole is partly responsible for the H-wave (Chapter 4), and sustained auricular systole is absent in fibrillation. If there are H-waves, they probably represent the headward force of the apex thrust. The pattern may be quite normal in the presence of fibrillation (Figure 116, *A*). This was first shown by Starr in 1941 (*3*). Sometimes a marked amplitude variation is observed from beat to beat; this is probably related to the irregular ventricular rate. In these circumstances the length of diastole (filling time) will be the factor limiting stroke volume (Figure 116, *C*). When the over-all amplitude is low and the pattern is very irregular in fibrillation, there is probably significant myocardial damage. This is a more frequent finding in fibrillation.

When myocardial damage becomes significant, even before there is frank clinical failure, the record becomes more abnormal and loses its regularity, definitiveness, and normal amplitude. In 1941 Starr (*3*) showed the increased ballistocardiogram abnormality when digitalis was stopped, with no apparent clinical change (Figure 117). Therefore, an abnormal irregular record in a rheumatic does not necessarily mean heart failure, but it implies more significant and serious disturbances than relatively uncomplicated valvular lesions. The patterns seen in failure are similar to those seen in failure from any cause, and have been discussed in Chapter 12. Starr has shown that improvement takes place in the pattern with digitalis (*3*), and this has been confirmed in our laboratory (Figure 118).

## REFERENCES

### RHEUMATIC HEART DISEASE

1. Starr, I.: "On the Clinical Characteristics of Patients with Subnormal Circulation in the Absence of Acute Heart Failure," *Tr. A. Am. Physicians,* **54**:163, 1939.

2. Starr, I., and Jonas, L.: "Syndrome of Subnormal Circulation in Ambulatory Patients," *Arch. Int. Med.,* **66**:1095, 1940.
3. Starr, I.: "Clinical Studies with the Ballistocardiograph," *Am. J. M. Sc.,* **202**:469, 1941.

CHAPTER FOURTEEN

# Miscellaneous Disorders

THE application of the ballistocardiogram in clinical medicine has been presented by categories, with selection of cases exemplifying the most common abnormalities. The section to be presented will deal with a variety of conditions in which the ballistocardiogram has been found to be of some use.

## 1. Pulmonary Disease

In many forms of pulmonary disease there occur changes which will interfere with normal circulation and which may produce an abnormal ballistocardiogram. The degree to which this occurs is dependent upon the type of pulmonary involvement and its extent.

### a. *Pulmonary Emphysema*

In these cases there are two factors which contribute to the pattern changes which generally consist of a markedly abnormal respiratory variation. Starr has reported increased amplitude in chronic pulmonary disease (*1* and *2*). This may reflect a compensatory mechanism. Because of the nature of the disease, the respiratory variation of the intrapleural pressure is increased—more negative pressures with inspiration, more positive pressures in the expiration (*2* and *3*). This pressure change probably accounts for the increased respiratory variation of the IJ stroke, as shown in Figure 119. The pattern may appear

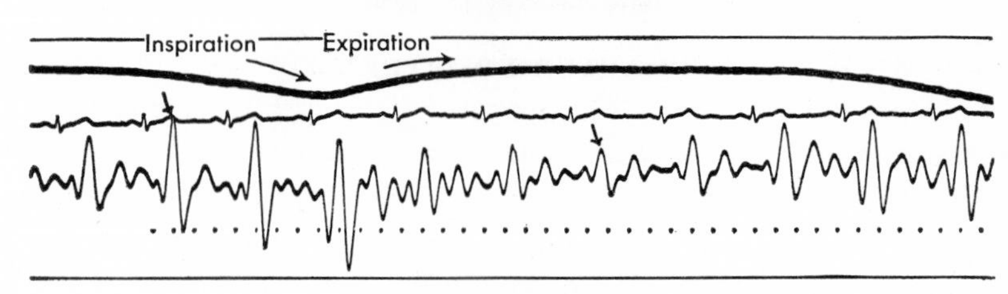


Pulmonary Emphysema

FIGURE 119. Note the increased respiratory variation. (Brown, H. R., Jr., and deLalla, V., Jr.: "The Ballistocardiogram, Description and Clinical Use," *Am. J. Med.,* **9**:718, 1950.)

quite irregular in pulmonary disease owing to tachypnea and dyspnea. Frequently, however, careful inspection will reveal distinct complexes.

b. *Silicosis*

In cases of silicosis both increased respiratory variation and abnormality of pattern have been noted as illustrated in Figure 120, *B*.

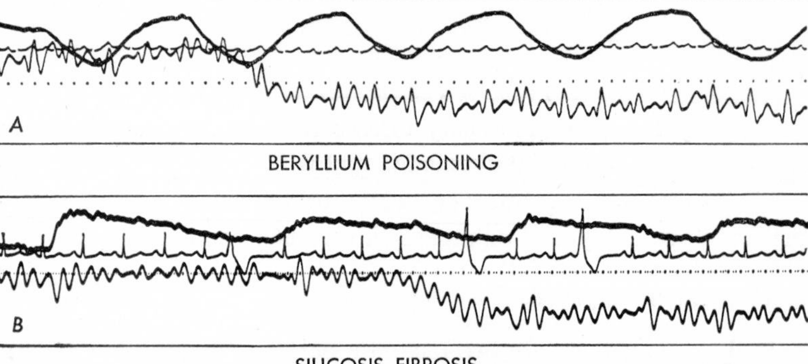


FIGURE 120. Tracing *A* shows a fairly normal pattern in a patient with beryllium pulmonary disease. *B* is a record of a male with silicosis and pulmonary fibrosis. Note the low amplitude and irregular expiratory patterns.

c. *Beryllium Poisoning*

A group of 9 cases of chronic beryllium poisoning was observed in this clinic; the oldest patient was 44 years. The trace shown in Figure

120, *A* was that of a 23-year-old woman who had had this disease for a period of 8 months. This record shows a slightly increased respiratory variation. This patient is in fairly good health, but 3 of the series of 9 have since died. The patterns of the more severely involved patients were so deranged by rapid and labored respirations that they were not reproduced.

d. *Pneumonectomy*

Increased amplitude of the ballistocardiogram has been observed after pneumonectomy by Starr (*1*). This is probably a compensatory mechanism.

**2. Metabolic Diseases**

Numerous diseases of the endocrine system have direct bearing upon body metabolism with changes in oxygen consumption and consequently cardiac output (*4*), and therefore, the amplitude of the ballistocardiogram.

a. *Hyperthyroidism*

Figure 121 shows a tracing of a 36-year-old man weighing but 112 lb, taken from Starr (*6*). There are increased stroke volume and in-

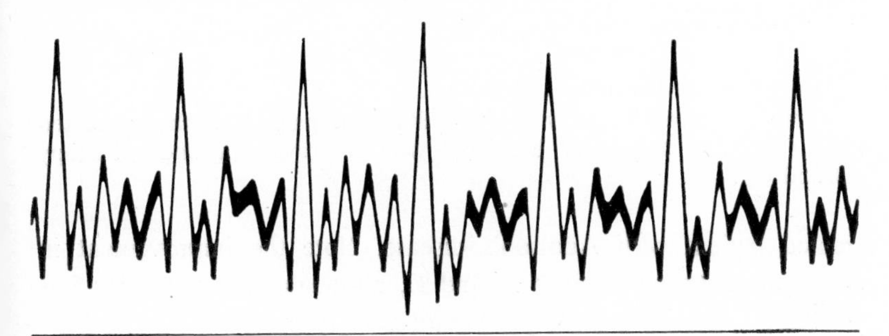

Thyrotoxicosis

FIGURE 121. A pattern of a hyperthyroid patient showing high output (large IJ strokes). (Starr, I., and Jonas, L.: "Supernormal Circulation in Resting Subjects (Hyperkinemia), with Study of Relation of Kinemic Abnormalities to Basal Metabolic Rate," *Arch. Int. Med.,* **71**:1, 1943.)

creased cardiac output over normal. The basal metabolic rate was plus 66 per cent.

b. *Hypothyroidism, Hypopituitarism, and Addison's Disease*

Figures 122 and 123 reproduce records showing the low amplitude that occurs with these diseases. Figure 122 shows serial traces on a

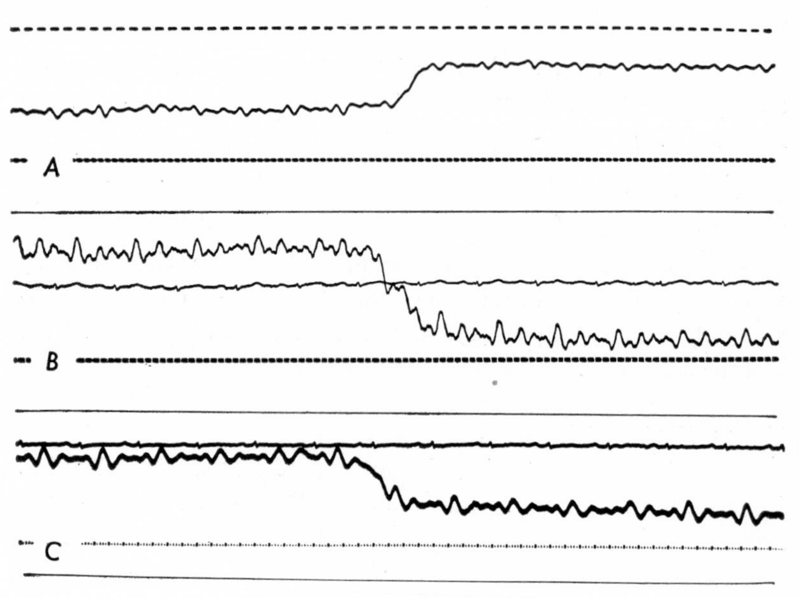


Endocrinopathy

FIGURE 122. Note the very low amplitude of pattern in the untreated state (*A*). The amplitude increased with improvement under therapy (*B* and *C*).

treated patient with Addison's disease. Note the improvement in amplitude between tracings *A* and *C*, although even with this improvement, the cardiac output is still very low.

### 3. Arteriovenous Aneurysm

There is a known increase in cardiac output associated with arteriovenous aneurysm to as much as 70 to 100 per cent over normal (*5*).

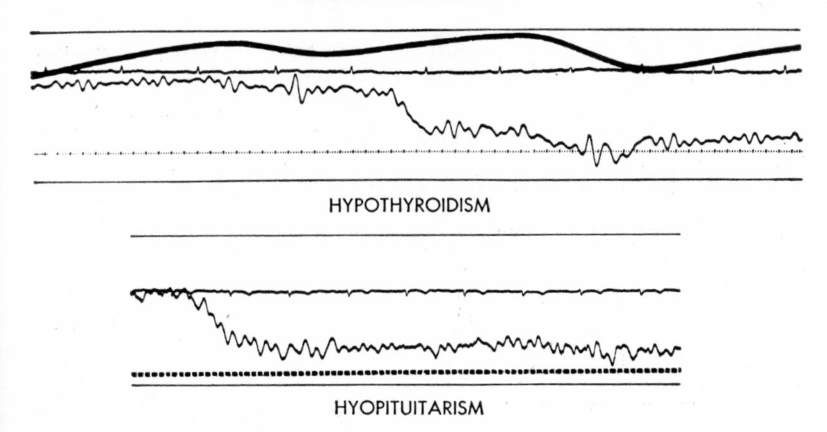


FIGURE 123. Note the low amplitudes corresponding to low cardiac output.

Figures 124 and 125 show two such cases (*5* and *6*). Note the reduced amplitude of the complexes upon cuff occlusion of the affected limb. Figure 126 is an example of moderately elevated stroke volume in a patient from our series with arteriovenous aneurysm.

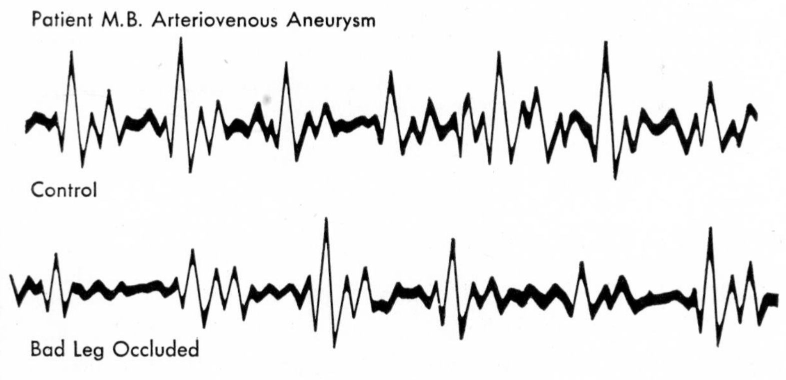


FIGURE 124. Traces taken before and after occlusion of an arteriovenous aneurysm. Note the diminished amplitude following occlusion. (Starr, I.: "Clinical Studies with the Ballistocardiogram," *Am. J. M. Sc.,* **202**:469, 1941.)

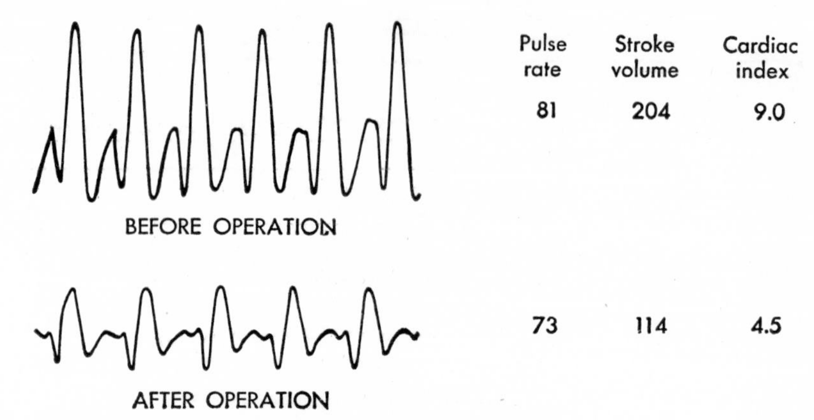


FIGURE 125. Low-frequency patterns showing diminished cardiac output following excision of an arteriovenous aneurysm. (Elkin, D. C., and Warren, J. V.: "Arterio-Venous Fistulas," *J.A.M.A.*, **134**:1524, 1947.)

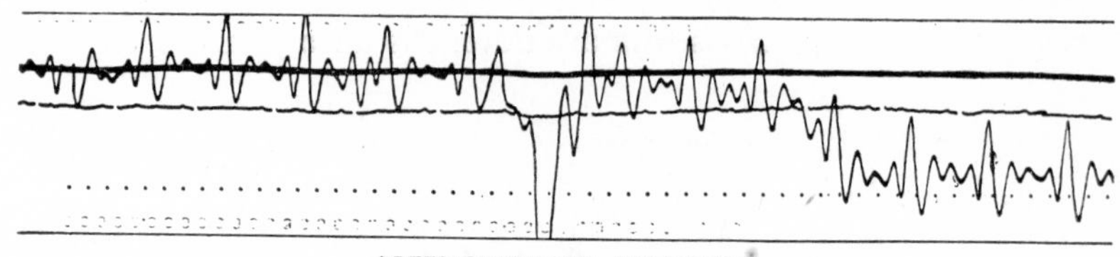


FIGURE 126. Young male with a femoral arteriovenous aneurysm. Note the large complexes indicating high output.

### 4. Record in 105-year-old Man

Figure 127 is the record obtained, just prior to his discharge, of a 105-year-old man who was admitted to the hospital for pneumonia. The fair degree of regularity and definitiveness of pattern is in keeping with his generally good cardiovascular condition for a person of such age.

### 5. Hypotension

Patterns associated with hypotension, both uncomplicated and of secondary nature, may be seen in Figure 128. The shallow to slurred K-waves are predominant features. In both traces *A* and *B*,

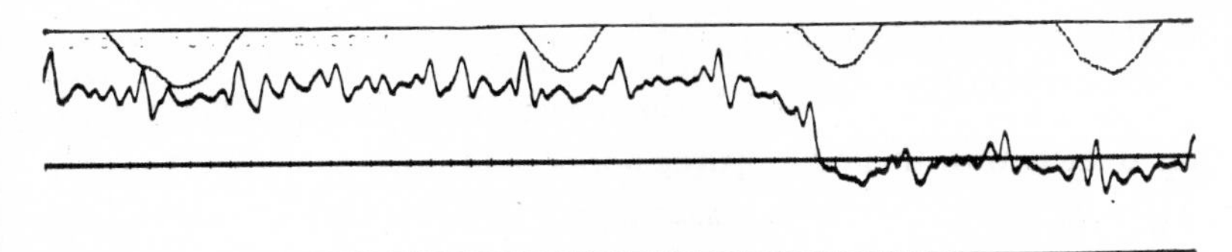


FIGURE 127. Record of a 105-year-old male showing fairly definite complexes, but with abnormal respiratory variation.

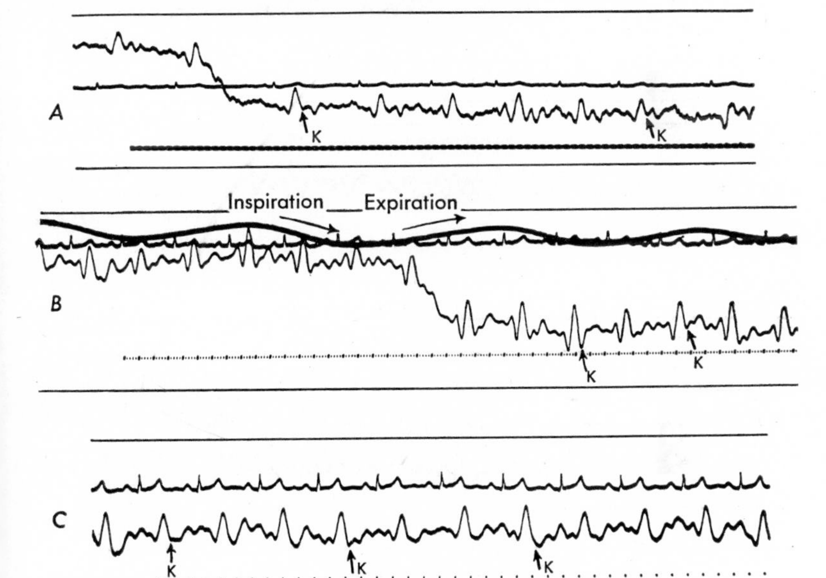


FIGURE 128. Records of three patients with hypotension. (*A*) A 13-year-old girl with anorexia nervosa. Note the shallow K-wave (arrow). (*B*) A 24-year-old woman who had chronic beryllium poisoning with minimal lung changes. Note the increase of K depth with inspiration. (*C*) A 19-year-old woman with congenital heart disease (probably patent interventricular septum). Note the changing shallow K valleys (arrows). (Trace *B* from Brown, H. R., Jr., and deLalla, V., Jr.: "The Ballistocardiogram, Description and Clinical Use," *Am. J. Med.*, **9**:718, 1950.)

shallow and plateaued K-waves similar to those seen in coarctation may be noted. The generally low wave complex amplitude is to be noted and is in keeping with low cardiac output.

## 6. Beriberi Heart Disease

A group of 3 patients with beriberi heart disease have been observed, all treated with thiamine hydrochloride and other vitamins, with recovery. Figure 129 shows a representative series of tracings obtained

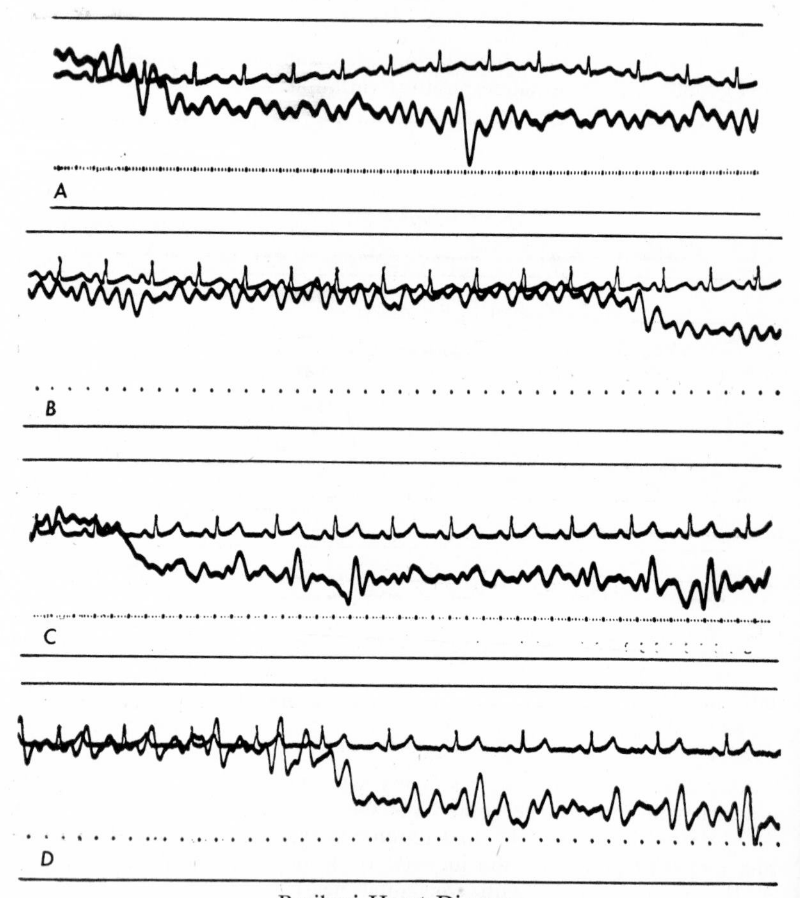


Beriberi Heart Disease

FIGURE 129. Serial tracings on a 28-year-old man who had beriberi heart disease. Note the improvement of the amplitude and pattern as the clinical picture improved with vitamin $B_1$ therapy. In tracing *A* (on admission) the pattern is low in amplitude, irregular and indefinite, and the H-K time is markedly variable. Tracing *D,* 1 month later, shows a more regular, definite pattern, improved amplitude, and a constant H-K time.

from 1 patient over a period of 30 days, with tracing *D* taken just prior to discharge. Note the general improvement in amplitude, regularity, and definitiveness of complexes. It is of interest that the H-K time, when measurable, appears to have increased with recovery.

## 7. Fever

The effect of a fever of 103.2°F induced artificially by killed typhoid baccilli inoculation is shown in Figure 130, taken from Starr

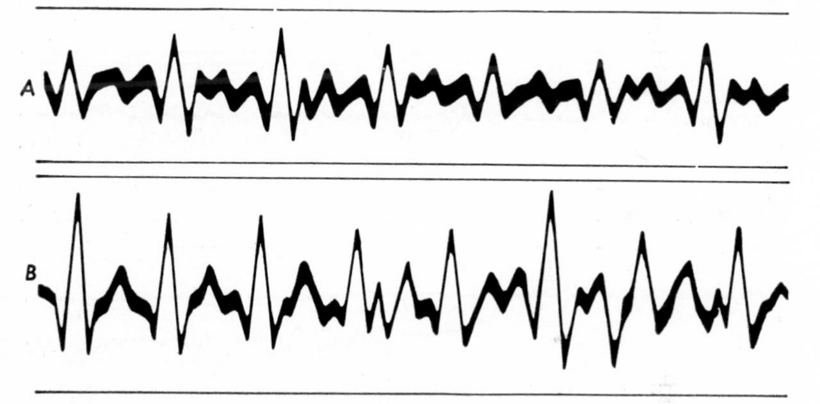


Effects of Fever

FIGURE 130. Note the increased amplitude in *B,* during fever, as contrasted to *A,* control. (Starr, I., and Jonas, L.: "Supernormal Circulation in Resting Subjects (Hyperkinemia), with Study of Relation of Kinemic Abnormalities to Basal Metabolic Rate," *Arch. Int. Med.,* **71**:1, 1943.)

(*6*). He states that the cardiac output in this man increased from 17 per cent above normal (control) to 79 per cent above normal (fever).

## 8. Heart Block

Figure 131 shows four examples of patients with complete heart block. The tendency toward long diastolic filling intervals and the good amplitude of the IJ strokes, particularly in *A, B,* and *D,* give some evidence why patients with complete heart block may do well

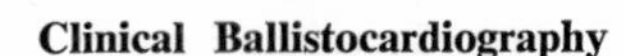

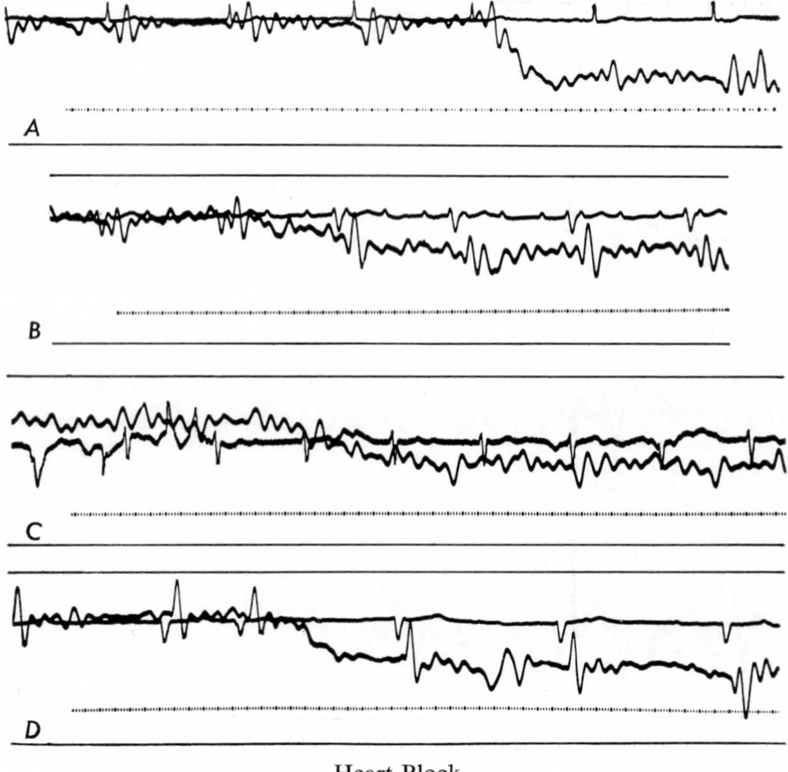


FIGURE 131. Four patients with complete heart block. Note the good amplitude in *B* and *D;* auricular ballistocardiogram complexes can be seen in *B,* following the P-waves of the electrocardiogram.

clinically. Such subjects show auricular ballistocardiogram complexes, as described in Chapter 4.

## 9. Tussive Syncope

Some interesting observations were noted in an adult male with tussive syncope of several years' duration. The effect of the Valsalva on the ballistocardiogram pattern may be seen in Figure 132, where tracing *A* is his resting pattern and *B* that obtained following Valsalva

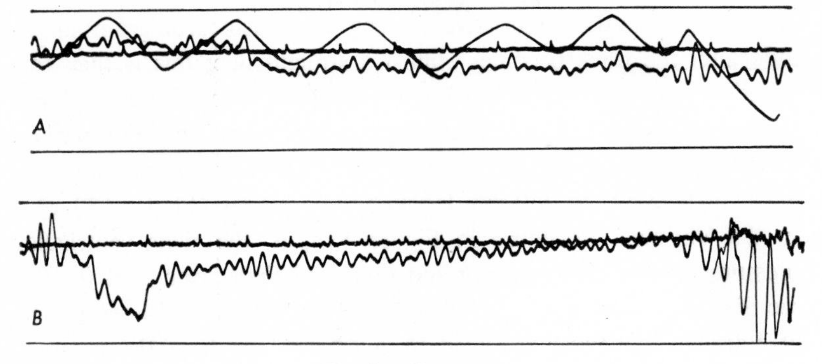


Tussive Syncope

FIGURE 132. Continuous record of a patient with tussive syncope taken just before and during a Valsalva maneuver. The onset of the Valsalva occurs at the beginning of the lower trace which is continuous with the upper record. Note the progressive diminution in amplitude as the Valsalva is held, finally ending in syncope and convulsions, occurring at the far right of the lower trace.

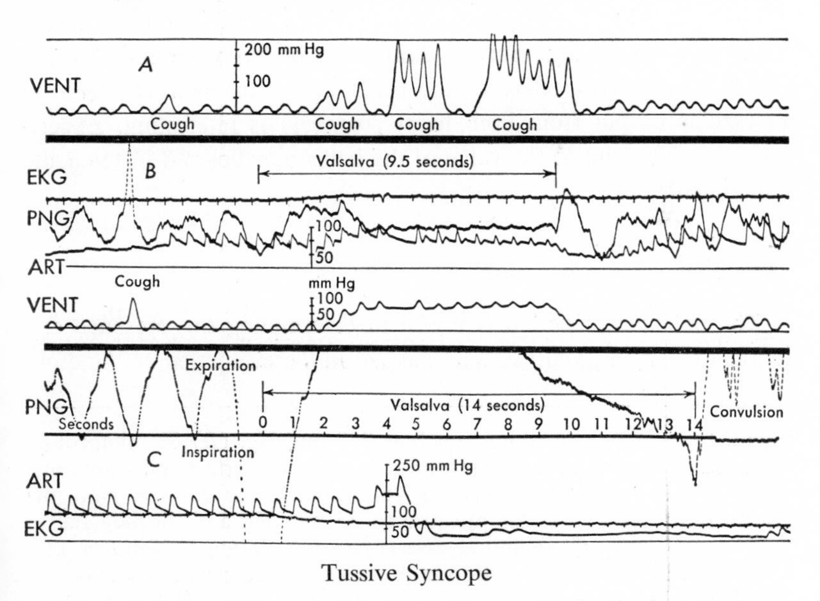


Tussive Syncope

FIGURE 133. Records of right ventricular and femoral artery pressures in a man with tussive syncope, during periods of coughing and Valsalva maneuvers. (*A*) Record of right ventricular pressure during coughing;

*(Caption continued on next page)*

maneuver. Note the progressive decrease in ballistocardiogram amplitude until the trace becomes almost a straight line; this is then followed by convulsive phenomena. Figure 133 gives further explanation as to the pathological physiology in this case. Note the marked increase in right ventricular pressure with coughing, the pressure rising as high as 225 to 240 mm Hg with the episodes (Figure 133, *A*). In the Valsalva procedure in Figure 133, *B*, the right ventricular pressure reached 100 mm Hg and remained there over 6 of the 9.5 sec that the breath was held. Tracing 133, *C*, shows a 14-sec period of Valsalva maneuver followed by a convulsion: here the pressure in the femoral artery rose from its normal pressure of 100 to 139 mm Hg to 210 and then fell to a low of 10 to 20 mm Hg, ending with convulsive episodes. The exact mechanism is not completely known, although the tussive phenomena and Valsalva procedures were thought by McCann (*7*) to cause pulmonary artery spasm, possibly in some reflex manner. It was suggested by deLalla (*8*) that the reduced venous return and exhaustion of pulmonary pool that occurs may be responsible for the marked diminution of left ventricular output and syncope. Irrespective of the exact cause, the marked decrease in cardiac output from both heart chambers is interesting. Experiments of this point to the value of the ballistocardiogram in the acute experiment.

## 10. Diphtheritic Myocarditis

The ballistocardiogram is useful in determining the presence and amount of any myocarditis and may aid in the evaluation of the diph-

---

note the rise in pressure to as much as 200 mm Hg. (*B*) Simultaneously recorded electrocardiogram, respirations, femoral artery pressure, and right ventricular pressure during a Valsalva held for 9.5 sec. Note the rise in the right ventricular pressure to 75 mm Hg and the late fall in arterial pressure. (*C*) Femoral artery pressure during a Valsalva held for 14 sec. Note the drastic drop in pressure, ending in syncope and convulsions at the fourteenth second. (McCann, W. S., Bruce, R. A., Lovejoy, F. W., Jr., Yu, P. N. G., Pearson, R., Emerson, G. B., Engel, G., and Kelly, J.: "Tussive Syncope," *Arch. Int. Med.*, **84**:845, 1949.)

theritic pattern. Figure 134 shows a trace of a patient with diphtheritic myocarditis.

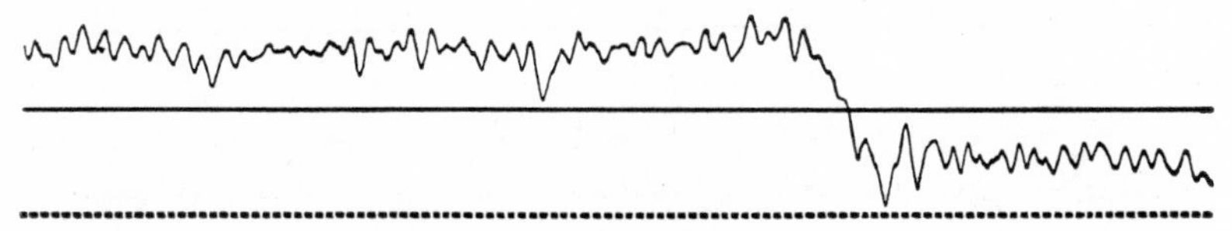

Diphtheritic Myocarditis

FIGURE 134. Record taken on an adult with diphtheritic myocarditis. Note the low amplitude and irregular complexes.

## 11. Neurocirculatory Asthenia

Starr has reported that abnormalities of amplitude of the ballistocardiogram pattern occur in patients with neurocirculatory asthenia (*9* and *10*). He states that either hyperkinemia (abnormally large cardiac output) or hypokinemia may occur, and that the symptomatology may reflect the inability of the circulation to adjust to changing demand. He studied a group of draftees who were diagnosed as having neurocirculatory asthenia. In 41 of the total of 58, the resting horizontal ballistocardiogram showed abnormally large complexes (*10*).

## 12. Congenital Heart Disease

The clinical value of the ballistocardiogram in congenital heart disease has thus far been limited to coarctation of the aorta in a specific sense, and to those anomalies which produce nonspecific changes in the ballistocardiogram such as may be seen with any interference with mechanical function. It is hoped that future work will bring to light other relationships.

In coarctation of the aorta the ballistocardiogram is useful in making the diagnosis (Figure 135) and in evaluating the postoperative state (Figure 136). The shallow K-wave that occurs with coarctation of the aorta was first mentioned by Hamilton (*11*). Since then

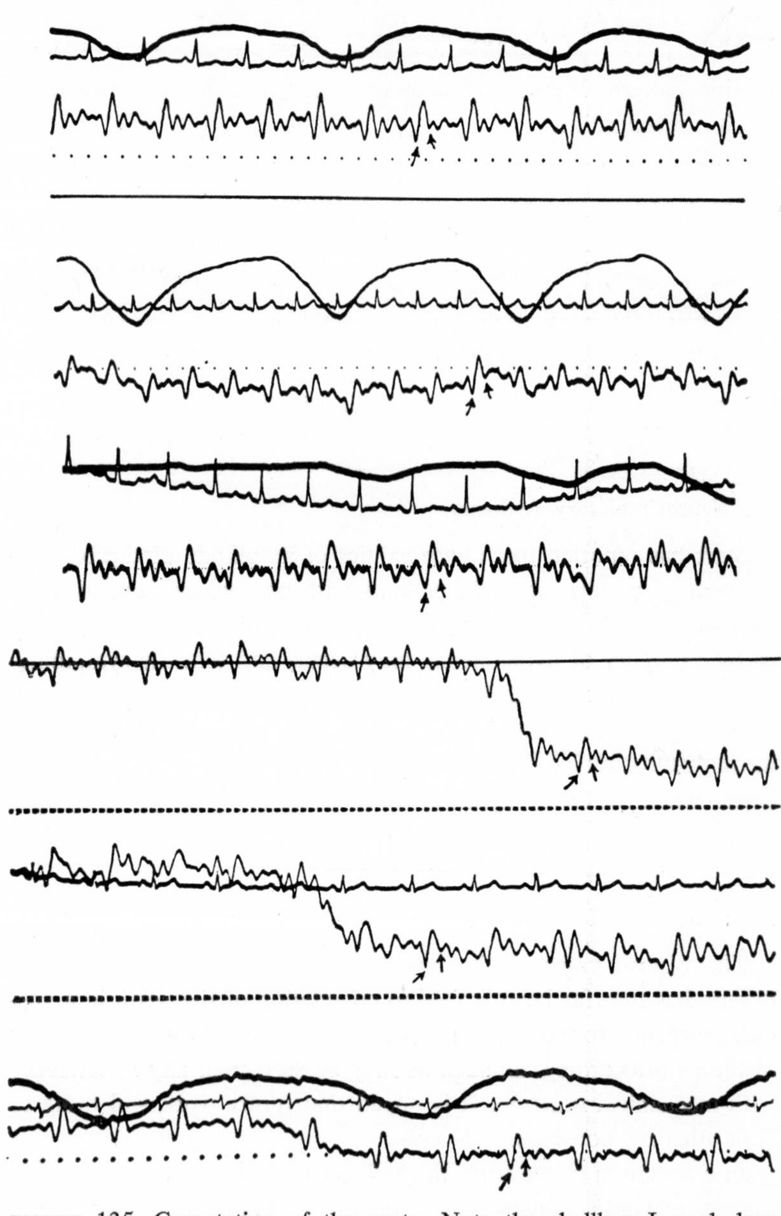

FIGURE 135. Coarctation of the aorta. Note the shalllow I- and deep K-waves (arrows). (Brown, H. R., Jr., Hoffman, M. J., and deLalla, V., Jr.: "Ballistocardiograms in Coarctation of the Aorta," *New England J. Med.,* **240**:175, 1949.)

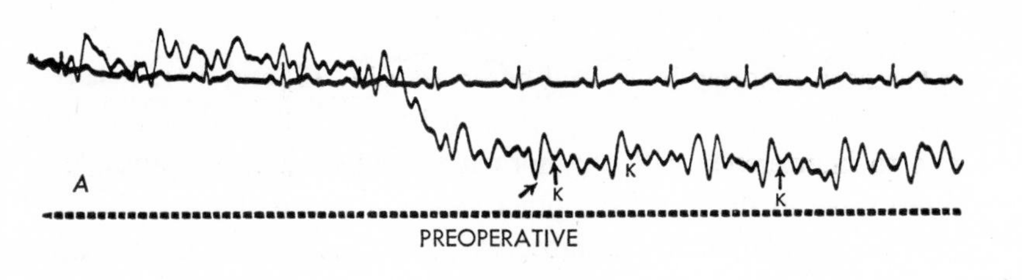


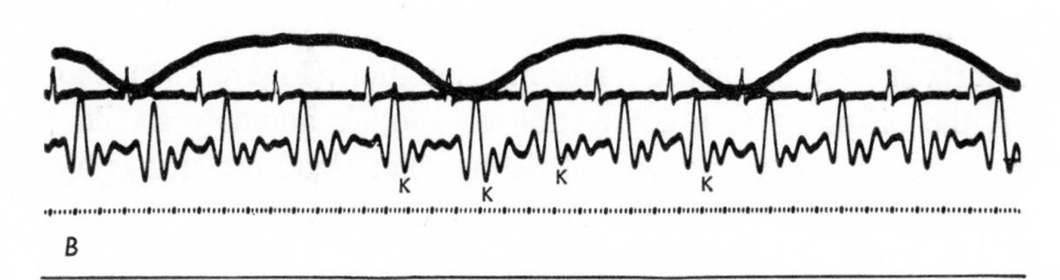


POSTOPERATIVE

Coarctation of the Aorta

FIGURE 136. Note the return of the I- and K-waves to normalcy following operation. (Brown, H. R., Jr., Hoffman, M. J., and deLalla, V., Jr.: "Ballistocardiograms in Coarctation of the Aorta," *New England J. Med.*, **240**:715, 1949.)

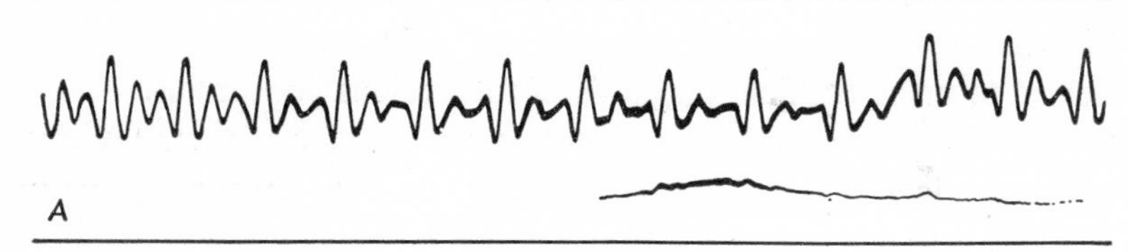


PREOPERATIVE

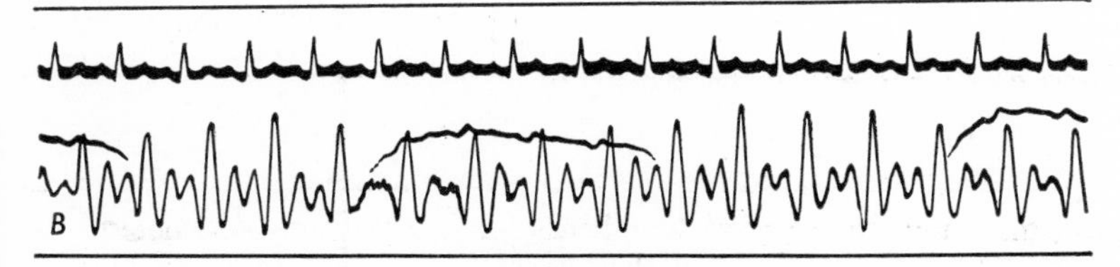


POSTOPERATIVE

Coarctation of the Aorta

FIGURE 137. Tracing *A* shows normal inspiratory K-waves in a patient with coarctation of the aorta; the expiratory K-waves are shallow. Compare with the K-waves in the postoperative tracing.

it has been reported by several observers (*11, 12,* and *13*). It is our opinion that the shallow K-wave seen in coarctation of the aorta is due to interference with the normal transmission of the aortic impulse wave to the legs. Any other situation that diminishes this impact on leg peripheral resistance will also produce shallow K-waves (i.e., aortic stenosis, hypotension, and very soft arterial walls such as in children). One of our series of 9 patients with coarctation of the aorta showed normal K-waves in inspiration (Figure 137). However, the diagnosis of a coarctation or another anomaly should be considered in this circumstance if the brachial blood pressure is high, since with a hypertension one expects a deep K-wave.

### 13. Pericarditis

Acute pericarditis may produce abnormalities in the ballistocardiogram pattern. Figure 138, *A,* shows a trace of a patient who at first was a diagnostic problem. Her complaints referred to the right upper quadrant where she also had spasm and tenderness. She had leukocytosis and fever; the very abnormal ballistocardiogram was the first objective evidence that incriminated the cardiovascular system and helped to make the final diagnosis of tuberculous pericarditis.

Constrictive pericarditis may reduce the cardiac output, thereby producing low amplitude of the IJ stroke. Starr has reported such a situation (*14*); Figure 138, *B* and *C,* shows pre- and postoperative ballistocardiogram patterns from a patient with constrictive pericarditis. Note the increased amplitude following operation.

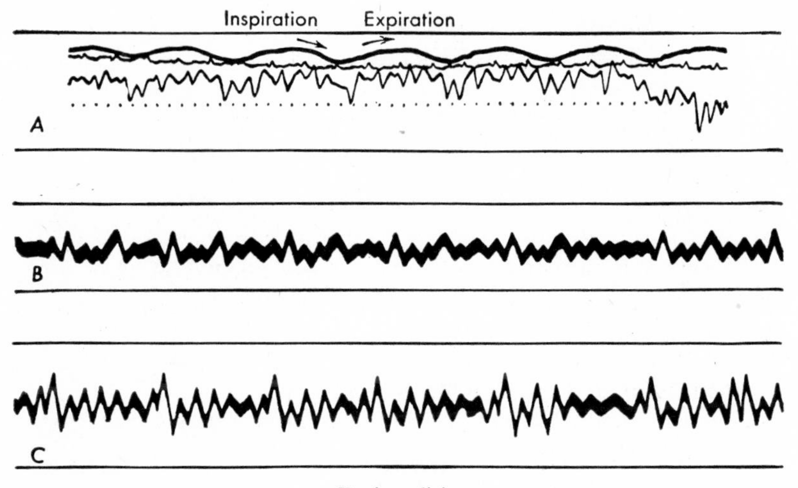


Pericarditis

FIGURE 138. (*A*) Record of a patient with acute tuberculous pericarditis. Note low amplitude and irregularity of pattern. *B* and *C* show the increased output following operation for constrictive pericarditis (*C*), as contrasted with the preoperative tracing (*B*). (Trace *A* from Brown, H. R., Jr., and deLalla V., Jr.: "The Ballistocardiogram, Description and Clinical Use," *Am. J. Med.*, **9**:718, 1950. Traces *B* and *C* from Starr, I., and Schroeder, H. A.: "Ballistocardiogram—Normal Standards, Abnormalities Commonly Found in Diseases of the Heart and Circulation, and Their Significance," *J. Clin. Investigation,* **19**:437, 1940.)

# REFERENCES

## MISCELLANEOUS DISORDERS


1. STARR, I.: "The Ballistocardiograph—an Instrument for Clinical Research and for Routine Clinical Diagnosis," *Harvey Lect.,* 1946–1947, Series 42, The Science Press, Lancaster, Pa., p. 194.
2. PAINE, J. R.: "Clinical Measurement of Pulmonary Elasticity," *J. Thoracic Surg.,* **9**:550, 1940.
3. DEAN, R. B., and VISSCHER, M. B.: "The Kinetics of Lung Ventilation," *Am. J. Physiol.,* **134**:450, 1941.
4. BROWN, H. R., JR., and PEARSON, R.: "Demonstration of a Positive Relationship between Cardiac Output and Oxygen Consumption," *Soc. Exp. Biol. Med.,* **65**:307, 1947.
5. ELKIN, D. C., and WARREN, J. V.: "Arterio-Venous Fistulas," *J.A.M.A.,* **134**:1524, 1947.
6. STARR, I., and JONAS, L.: "Supernormal Circulation in Resting Subjects (Hyperkinemia), with Study of Relation of Kinemic Abnormalities to Basal Metabolic Rate," *Arch. Int. Med.,* **71**:1, 1943.
7. MCCANN, W. S., BRUCE, R. A., LOVEJOY, F. W., JR., YU, P. N. G., PEARSON, R., EMERSON, G. B., ENGEL, G., and KELLY, J.: "Tussive Syncope," *Arch. Int. Med.,* **84**:845, 1949.
8. DELALLA, V., JR., and BROWN, H. R., JR.: "The Respiratory Variation of the Ballistocardiogram," *Am. J. Med.,* **9**:728, 1950.
9. STARR, I.: "Abnormalities of the Amount of Circulation (Hyper and Hypokinemia) and Their Relation to Neurocirculatory Asthenia and Kindred Diagnosis," *Am. J. M. Sc.,* **204**:573, 1942.
10. STARR, I.: "Ballistocardiographic Studies of Draftees Rejected for Neurocirculatory Asthenia," *War Med.,* **5**:155, 1944.
11. HAMILTON, W. F., REMINGTON, J. W., and DOW, P.: "Relationship between Cardiac Ejection Curve and Ballistocardiographic Forces," *Am. J. Physiol.,* **144**:557, 1945.
12. BROWN, H. R., JR., HOFFMAN, M. J., and DELALLA, V., JR.: "Ballistocardiograms in Coarctation of the Aorta," *New England J. Med.,* **240**:715, 1949.
13. NICKERSON, J. L., HUMPHREYS, G. H., DETERLING, R. A., FLEMING, T. C., and MATERS, J. A. L.: "Diagnosis of Coarctation with the Aid of the Low Frequency, Critically Damped Ballistocardiograph," *Circulation,* **1**:1032, 1950.

14. MURPHY, R. A.: "Ballistocardiographic Patterns in Intraluminal Aortic Obstructions," *Am. Heart J.*, **39**:174, 1950.
15. STARR, I., and SCHROEDER, H. A.: "Ballistocardiogram—Normal Standards, Abnormalities Commonly Found in Diseases of the Heart and Circulation, and Their Significance," *J. Clin. Investigation*, **19**:437, 1940.

# INDEX